CONQUER DEPRESSION NOW

From Sad to Glad at Home, School, and Work

By David Wiesenberg

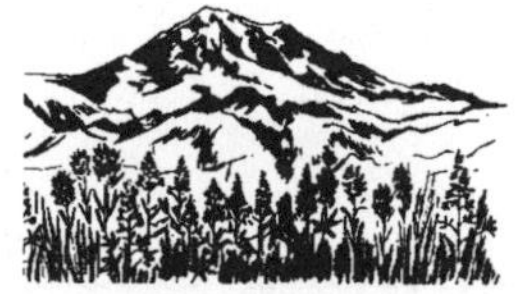

Meadow Mountain Press

CONQUER DEPRESSION NOW

From Sad to Glad at Home, School, and Work

By David Wiesenberg

Published by:

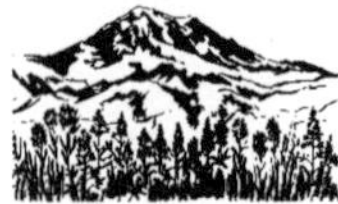

Meadow Mountain Press
1375 Coney Island Avenue • Suite 136 • Brooklyn • NY 11230
Tel. (718) 338 1559 • Fax. (718) 258-4566

==================================

Publisher's Cataloging-in-Publication Data

Wiesenberg, David S., 1954—
Conquer Depression Now: From Sad to Glad at Home, School, and Work / David S. Wiesenberg. — 1st ed.
p. cm.
Includes bibliographical references and index.
ISBN 0-9647692-5-5
1. Depression, Mental. 2. Psychology, Pathological.
3. Self-actualization (Psychology). I. Title
RC537 1995
616.852'7—dc20 95-94635

Library of Congress Catalog Card Number: 95-94635
ISBN 0-9647692-5-5: $14.95 Softcover
Cover design and illustration by Lightbourne Images copyright © 1996
Printed by Gilliland Printing, Inc., on 100% recycled, acid-free paper
Printed in the United States of America

What others are saying about this book:

An outstanding guide for the layman in readable language.
Richard Balon, M.D.,
director of medical student education in psychiatry,
Wayne State University, Detroit, Michigan.

A must for all managers interested in the mental health and productivity of their employees. Well organized, clear and helpful.
Maurice Askinazi,
systems administrator,
Internal Revenue Service.

Easy to read and accessible; good for both people who are suffering ***and*** *their companions. I like the analogy between physical and mental illness so that sufferers will stop blaming themselves and seek help.*
Sally Morrison,
former mid-Suffolk president,
National Organization for Women.

Depression is no laughing matter—that's why I'm very pleased and proud that my "POT-SHOTS" cartoons were chosen to illustrate this important work, which I hope will be of great help to many people.
Ashleigh Brilliant,
author of "I feel Much Better Now That I've Given Up Hope."

Clear, dependable approach to overcoming depression that the average reader will find very useful and empowering.
Sandy Eckstein, M.S.W.,
social worker, Passaic, New Jersey.

No more interminable sessions with incompetent shrinks with the no-nonsense advice given in this book!
Marty Martinez, WNEW-FM 102.7,
producer and host of "FM—Magazine of the Airways."

TABLE OF CONTENTS

TABLE OF CONTENTS

PART THREE: OVERCOMING DEPRESSION

PART FOUR: REFERENCES AND SOURCES

Foreword

Churchill called it "the black dog." The early Greek physicians labeled it "melancholie," which approximately translates as "black bile." Being neither statesman nor Greek, I call it "depression." The National Depressive and Manic-Depressive Association has a mission to spread public awareness of this medical illness, foster self-help for patients and families, eliminate discrimination and stigma, and improve the availability and quality of help and support. This book goes a long way in helping to achieve that goal and dream. It is a trustworthy, quality guide for the effective management of depression that is easy to read. I only wish I had had it as a resource to speed my own recovery from the periods of depression I used to go through.

Both people who feel depressed and their friends and relatives will find it useful. I regret that I never had the patience to write as thorough an information resource. Authors who are mental health professionals unwittingly omit large areas of information essential to a patient. David Wiesenberg's particular contribution to the self-help/patient information library stems from his personal experience and insight. As it were, he fills in the blanks.

David Wiesenberg clearly explains depression and presents the practical problems which every depressed person must face. Unique among the "self-help" genre, the emphasis here is on the practical, the do-able and the real. This is an overview of depression, the available types of treatment, and the resources needed for the proper resolution of this condition. David Wiesenberg discusses the several biochemical causes for depression. He covers its aftermath in which faulty patterns of depressed thinking persist. He establishes high standards in his honest coverage of how to select and where to find the treatment of choice, what to expect in terms of satisfaction, and financial matters. An excellent series of resources will widen the availability of medications, mental health professionals, self-help groups, and low-cost/free care for many readers.

FRANK BURGMANN
President, National Depressive and Manic-Depressive Association

Preface

My beloved wife died of illness at the young age of 28 years. After her death I fell into depression, which went on and on for years and would not clear up. However, the doctors in England, where I was living at the time, did not pick up on the fact that I was ill. Had they diagnosed the illness and treated it, I would never have written this book.

In 1990 I moved to New York. December is an exciting month for most people, preparing for and enjoying the holidays, the celebrations, and the bringing in of the new year. At that time I felt anything but happy; in fact, I wished I were dead and free from the burden of life. To tell the truth, I used to consider ways of committing suicide but did not have the guts to do it!

That month I traveled up to Rochester for a meeting. In those days I rarely read the newspapers but I decided to buy a copy of the "New York Times" because the train journey would last for over seven hours and I had nothing to do. Buried deep among the inside pages was an advertisement entitled "Do You Feel Depressed?" offering participation in a free treatment study at the Columbia-Presbyterian Medical Center in Manhattan.

Was I depressed? I wondered. Odd though it sounds, I found it hard to work out the answer. Since I had long forgotten the feeling and meaning of "happiness," I thought my state of mind was "normal." In fact, what did "depressed" actually mean?

Still, the Columbia-Presbyterian Medical Center was a reputable institution and the treatment study was free so there was no harm in trying it out. After completing lengthy questionnaires and detailed interviews, I was informed that my diagnosis indicated a severe depression. However, Steven Donovan, M.D. (a conscientious doctor under whose care I was), was confident it could be treated successfully. I could join the treatment study which concerned the (then) new drug Prozac. The illness made me how I felt, and it was all due to neurotransmitter malfunctioning in the brain.

At first I did not believe Dr. Donovan. I could not see how a malady of the mind and mood could have a physical cause. Like many others, I thought the only antidote to depression lay in "thinking positive." In the treatment study I took a daily dose of Prozac and my mood began to lift. After four months my mood suddenly plunged uncontrollably and inexplicably, and I was in danger of making a suicide attempt. Nothing like that had ever happened to me before. Doctor Donovan investigated and found that the medicine had been changed to an ineffective placebo for the previous month without our knowledge.

That was the point of the study: if a patient recovered with Prozac, would he (she) relapse by discontinuing. In my case, I certainly did! Dr. Donovan explained it was the best news I could have. It meant most definitely that my depression **was** due to neurotransmitter malfunctioning, and that Prozac would work for me and make me better. It was only then that I believed that depression had a physical cause.

Half the people who take Prozac experience unpleasant side effects. Fortunately, I was not one of them. I never had any side effects to complain about. As far as I was concerned, I could have been taking vitamin pills.

As I slowly recovered, I discovered how common this illness is, how it affects over 10% of the population, and how easily treatable it is once it is correctly diagnosed. Unfortunately, less than one in three family doctors diagnose and/or treat it properly. That is why the illness is so prevalent, lingers on, and is widely misunderstood. It saps people of their vitality, and disguises their "true personality." It accounts for billions of dollars lost at work, since it is the cause of poor productivity, prolonged absenteeism, and industrial accidents.

I do not wish the millions of people with depression to suffer needlessly as I did. Nor do I like to see industrial competitiveness blunted by an easily treatable illness. I look forward to the day (which I predict will be perhaps within five years, certainly within ten) when depression will no longer be a scourge and the stigma surrounding it will be a thing of the past. The same happened to cholera and diphtheria in the nineteenth century and polio in the 1950s after effective treatments were found. Depression can be diagnosed and treated effectively at onset; no one needs to suffer for nothing.

All that is needed is for the public to be well-informed about this illness, know where to go when one has it, be aware of the treatments available, and understand how to monitor recovery. It is with the aim of helping to achieve this dream and goal that I have written this book.

DAVID WIESENBERG

A Request to the Reader

One of the major problems facing a person with depression who is seeking treatment is knowing where to find a good mental health practitioner. Unfortunately, there are far too many people who suffer needlessly while spending a lot of time and money receiving poor or improper treatment.

In order to give confidence to those seeking treatment for the first time, I would like to compile a list of mental health practitioners with whom people have had good experiences. Please write to me (℅ Meadow Mountain Press, 1375 Coney Island Avenue, #136, Brooklyn, NY 11230) and share your experiences of practitioners you would like to recommend and why. Your personal details will be held in strict confidentiality.

Please include: the name, address and profession of the practitioner; the nature of the illness; and the type, length, cost and effectiveness of treatment, how well it was discussed, if and how it was monitored, etc.

Lastly, the information in this book has been carefully checked and is correct to the best of my knowledge as of January 1996. Nevertheless, in a work of this length it is virtually impossible to eliminate all errors and, as time goes by, some information may change. If you find any such inaccuracies, please would you let me know so that I can update and improve future editions of this book.

Acknowledgments

Thanks are due to the many people, authorities, and sources who have contributed to the writing and preparation of this book.

Gratitude is expressed to the following medical experts who each generously gave of their time in reviewing part or all of the book: Richard Balon, M.D. (Associate Professor of Psychiatry and Director of Medical Student Education in Psychiatry at Wayne State University, Michigan); Robert Boland, M.D. (Assistant Professor of Psychiatry at Brown University School of Medicine, Providence, Rhode Island, and committee member of the Centers for Disease Control and Prevention in Atlanta); Hugo Van Dooren, M.D., P.S. (Clinical Professor at the University of Washington School of Medicine, and Medical Director of the Mental Health Unit, Puget Sound Hospital, Tacoma, Washington); Glen R. Elliott, M.D. (Associate Professor and Director of Child and Adolescent Psychiatry at the University of California at San Francisco School of Medicine); William A. Florio, M.D. (psychiatrist in private practice, Brooklyn, New York); and finally Thomas W. Uhde, M.D. (Professor and Chairman, Department of Psychiatry, Wayne State University, Michigan).

The following people were invaluable in providing lay reviews: Kathy and Maurice Askinazi, James Besser, Sandy Eckstein, Ann Helfgott, Nancy Jakubowyc, Esther Mandel, Sally Morrison, and Jay Neinstein. Appreciation is due to Joyce Gottlieb, book committee member of the National Depressive and Manic-Depressive Association, who received the manuscript enthusiastically and introduced me to Frank Burgmann, president of that organization, who kindly agreed to write the foreword. Herbert E. Klein, editor and publisher of "Psychotherapy Finances," provided interesting insights into the costs of treatment for depression.

Tribute must be paid to the valiant government employees in the National Institutes of Health who put themselves out to provide current research data despite pressure caused by the enormous backlog of work resulting from the office shutdowns that occurred during the budget impasse between Congress and President Clinton. Bob Silberfarb, Marie Parker, and Nazli Haq have been very helpful in this respect.

The humorous "Pot-Shot" illustrations, reprinted by permission of Ashleigh Brilliant Enterprises, have been invaluable in lightening up the atmosphere of the book and will undoubtedly help cheer up a lot of people with depression. They are extracted from the books "I Feel Much Better Now That I've Given Up Hope" and "We've Been Through So Much Together And Most of It Was Your Fault," authored by Ashleigh Brilliant.

Shannon Bodie who works for Lightbourne Images, the cover designer and illustrator, posed for the photograph on the front cover. She symbolizes a person looking out hopefully from a gloomy present to a bright and inviting future.

Last but not least, my parents and family are thanked for encouraging me to persevere and complete the task at hand.

I sincerely thank all these fine people and know they are proud of their contribution to the success of this work.

Warning and Disclaimer

The information in this book is designed to supplement, not substitute for, the advice and directions of a trained medical professional. It is sold with the understanding that the author and publisher are not engaged in rendering psychiatric, financial, legal, or other professional services. This book should not be used as a manual of self-diagnosis or self-treatment. All matters regarding your health require medical supervision; you should always consult with your own physician before starting or making changes in any medical treatment, diet, exercise, or other health program. The author and publisher will have neither liability nor responsibility to any person or entity with respect to any loss or damage caused, or alleged to be caused, directly or indirectly by the information contained in this book.

If you do not wish to be bound by the above, you may return this book to the publisher for a full refund.

PART ONE:

INTRODUCTION

Chapter 1

What is Depression?

Yes, what exactly **is** depression? Everyone feels sad from time to time. That is life, isn't it? So when is feeling blue perfectly normal and when is it something to worry about?

Unfortunately, there is no clear cut answer. It really depends on your intuition. Is your sadness so deep or so prolonged that it is interfering with your life? That is the basic question you ask yourself. If the answer is "yes," then, yes, it is something to worry about.

Now, wouldn't it be much simpler if depression was an illness like a broken leg? If you were worried about having a broken leg, all you have to do is go and have an x-ray. You will soon know one way or another. Either your leg is broken or it is not. That's all there is to it.

POT-SHOTS NO. 4459.
I AM TRYING VERY HARD TO FUNCTION
IN A HOSTILE ENVIRONMENT CALLED "LIFE".
©ASHLEIGH BRILLIANT 1988. Ashleigh Brilliant

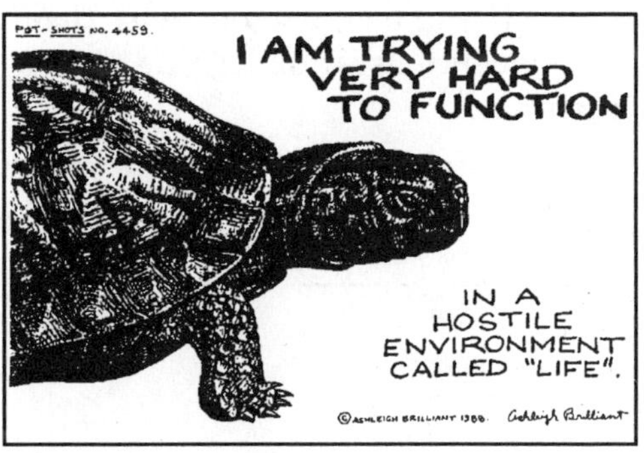

Depression is more like having a cold, or a headache, or pimples on the skin. Imagine you have a cold. Your throat is sore, you cough a lot, and your nose is running. You feel uncomfortable. So you take aspirin, suck lozenges, and wait. If you feel better after a few days, and you do not catch another cold for several weeks, then you have nothing to worry about.

On the other hand, if the cold will just not go away, and you have had a fever, a sore throat, and a runny nose for three weeks, what do you do then? Alternatively, if you have been catching colds every week for the last three months, do you shrug it off cheerfully and forget about it? Of course not! Something is very wrong and it is time to see your doctor. Perhaps you have influenza or even pneumonia.

Suppose you have a headache. You take an aspirin and go to bed. The headache should be gone the next morning; certainly in a day or two. On the other hand, if it goes on for many days, or it becomes so painful that you cannot bear it, the next step is clear: a trip to your doctor. Maybe you have a migraine.

Similarly with a pimple on the skin. Just a little red spot. Could be acne. Or a tiny boil. Should clear in few days. But if it does not, or you get more spots and they spread all over your body, then it is time to get help. You probably have the measles!

It's the same with depression. Depression should lift within a few hours or days. It does for most people. On the other hand, if it lasts more than about two weeks, then it is no longer normal and it is perfectly proper to seek help from the doctor. Alternatively, if it becomes so intense that it stops you getting on with your life properly, then it is time to put your doctor to work. In fact, it would be foolish to sit back and do nothing!

If you feel blue for more than two weeks, or so sad that you cannot concentrate on leading your life properly, then seek medical attention.

> *Tough times never last, but tough people do.*
>
> Robert Schuller (1926–)

Chapter 2

Types of Depression

Depression belongs to the family of illnesses called affective disorders. ("Affective" is a psychological term which means "pertaining to feeling or emotion.") Another type of affective disorder is mania. There are two main types of depression:

1. **Major depression.** The more severe form characterized by an inability to cheer up for short periods
2. **Dysthymia.** Mild, chronic depression

Based on these may be the following patterns and variations:

3. **Double depression.** Major depression coinciding with dysthymia
4. **Atypical depression.** Characterized by too much sleep and appetite rather than too little, and an ability to cheer up for short periods
5. **Psychotic depression.** Severe form with delusions and/or hallucinations
6. **Seasonal affective disorder (SAD).** Depression experienced during only the winter
7. **Postpartum depression.** Experienced by mothers shortly after giving birth
8. **Involutional depression.** Experienced by the elderly
9. **Reactive depression.** Appears in response to an external event
10. **Endogenous depression.** Comes out of the blue without apparent cause

Mania is an exaggerated feeling of well-being, the opposite of depression. Depression and mania may also follow each other in cycles. Although popularly known as manic depression, psychiatrists prefer to call this condition "bipolar disorder" or "bipolar depression."

(Depression by itself is termed "unipolar disorder" or "unipolar depression.") There are also patterns and variations:

11. **Bipolar I.** Episodes of severe depression and severe mania
12. **Hypomania.** A mild form of mania
13. **Bipolar II.** Episodes of severe depression and hypomania
14. **Cyclothymia.** Chronic, mild episodes of depression and mania
15. **Rapid cycling.** Where moods alternate very frequently

Note that a person can suffer from several types of depression at the same time. Strange though it sounds, it is even possible to have symptoms of depression and mania at the same time! This is called a "mixed pattern."

People are often confused by the terms "major" and "atypical" depression. A comparison is shown in following table:

DIFFERENCES BETWEEN MAJOR AND ATYPICAL DEPRESSION

Feature	Major	Atypical
Occurrence	About equally common among people	
Intensity	Can be very severe with risk of suicide; equally serious	
Appetite	Decreased	Increased
Sleep	Disturbed	Excessive
Worst time of day	Morning	Evening
Duration	Well-defined episodes	Tends to be continuous
Other common features (not always present)	Inability to be cheered up by anything	Extreme sensitivity to rejection; craving for sweet foods; ability to cheer up temporarily

Our greatest glory is not in never failing, but in rising every time we fail.

Confucius (551–479 B.C.)

Chapter 3

Biological Origin of Depression

All healthy people experience brief periods of depression from time to time. This is perfectly natural. Often depression is set off by an extremely upsetting event. Failing an important examination, going bankrupt and losing a close relative are common examples. This depression is said to be reactive, that is, caused by external circumstances. Time and counseling are the best healers for this kind of depression and there is no need for medical treatment unless the depression is prolonged and severe.

©ASHLEIGH BRILLIANT 1986.
POT-SHOTS NO. 4600.
WHICH DO I NEED MORE ~
TO PULL MYSELF TOGETHER,
OR TO LET MYSELF GO?
Ashleigh Brilliant

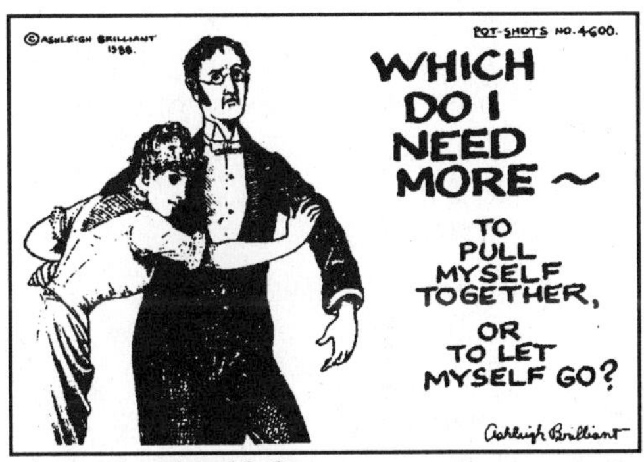

Another type of depression affects about one in ten people sometime in their lives. Although it may be triggered off by a relatively minor sad event which most people manage to take in their stride, the depression tends to be unusually severe or long lasting. Sometimes it comes about by itself for no apparent reason without any external event taking place. This type of depression is said to be endogenous, that is, caused by internal circumstances.

All depression, both reactive and endogenous, reflects a biochemical imbalance in the brain. Many people erroneously believe that mild or reactive depression is merely a matter of sad thoughts that can be "talked out of" with psychotherapy and has nothing to do with the brain chemistry. At the same time, they see serious, major depression as a direct result of biochemical malfunctioning in the brain which requires medical drugs to fix. In their opinion, mild depression cannot be helped with drugs and major depression cannot be helped with psychotherapy.

The truth is that the thoughts of the mind affect the chemistry in the brain and vice versa. Therefore, medical drugs may be used to treat mild depression (and are often very effective for it). In theory psychotherapy also helps alleviate major depression. In practice, however, the depression is usually so deep that the patient has lost the motivation and attention required to absorb the psychotherapeutic treatment.

Another common misconception is that depression has nothing to do with any other illness. This is not true; a few illnesses cause depression as one of their symptoms. Most people with flu experience a low, miserable time which clears up as the illness passes away. This is nothing to be alarmed about. Unfortunately, a few people are afflicted by illnesses which can produce long-term depression and need medical attention. These illnesses include:

1. Alcoholism
2. Cardiovascular disorders, e.g., congestive heart failure
3. Encephalopathy
4. Endocrine and metabolic disorders, e.g.:
   (a) Addison's disease
   (b) Cushing's disease
   (c) diabetes
   (d) hyperthyroidism
   (e) hypothyroidism
   (f) porphyria
5. Gastrointestinal disorders, e.g., ulcerative colitis
6. Hematological disorders, e.g., anemia
7. Infectious diseases, e.g.:
   (a) AIDS
   (b) hepatitis
   (c) influenza
   (d) mononucleosis
   (e) syphilis
   (f) tuberculosis
8. Malignancies (cancer)
9. Menopause
10. Multiple sclerosis
11. Nutritional disorders

12. Respiratory disorders, e.g.:
    (a) chronic obstructive pulmonary disease
    (b) asthma
13. Rheumatoid arthritis
14. Uremia

Certain drugs used to treat serious illnesses produce side effects which are the cause of depression. Many people are unaware that valium and similar drugs for anxiety actually **increase** depression. So does alcohol. Unfortunately, many people with mild depression take anti-anxiety drugs or drink alcohol to drown their sorrows. Not only do they cause addiction, they actually worsen the depression. Once the effect of the drugs or drink wears off, the patient feels even worse and wants to take more. Consequently, a vicious circle is born.

Below is a list of some of the drug types that may cause depression in some people. If you are taking any of them and you have been feeling depressed for a considerable time, discuss with your doctor whether the drug could be the cause and whether he (she) could replace it with another. For a full list of drugs, see References and Sources (page 157).

DRUGS THAT MAY CAUSE DEPRESSION

	Type of drug
1.	Anti-anxiety drugs
2.	Antihypertensives (to treat high blood pressure)
3.	Antiparkinsonism drugs
4.	Corticosteroids
5.	Hormones
6.	Oral contraceptives

As can be seen, many kinds of illnesses and drugs may cause depression. Therefore, a careful physical examination is important when seeking treatment.

Most people are reading this book because they are feeling depressed or because they know someone who is feeling depressed. They want to do something about it and are looking for answers. Knowing the biological cause is not a solution, and those who are not scientifically minded may skip the rest of this section if they like. However, those who are and would like to satisfy their curiosity should read on.

The human brain, which even today scientists do not fully understand, contains billions of nerve cells. (Some say that there are as many nerve cells in the brain as there are stars in the galaxy!) These are interconnected in an enormously sophisticated network. Each cell can send messages to another through the network by means of tiny electrical currents.

It is somewhat similar to a huge network of telephone exchanges. The "telephone exchanges" of the brain are called neurons and the "wires" are called axons. But there is an important difference. In a telephone exchange the wires touch each other directly. In the brain, however, the nerve axons do not quite touch each other. The synapse, a small gap filled with liquid (synaptic fluid) lies in between. Electrical messages are transferred to tiny carriers (neurotransmitters) which flow across the gap where they are taken up by cellular receptors. Without these carriers, the messages could not travel from nerve cell to nerve cell. This is schematically illustrated in figure 1 ("Brain nerve cells") and figure 2 ("Chemical messengers flowing between brain nerve endings").

There are several kinds of neurotransmitters, the most well-known of which are called serotonin, norepinephrine, and dopamine. About twenty-four have been discovered to date but scientists believe there may be several hundred.

Normally, there is an ample supply of neurotransmitters to carry messages from one brain cell to another. For some reason which is not yet known, scientists have discovered that a person's mood becomes affected when there is an imbalance of these carriers. (This may sound odd. After all, what can message carriers have to do with mood? Yet, somehow they do.)

Recent research indicates mood changes are also caused by receptor changes and malfunctioning of the interaction between the neurotransmitters and receptors. (This has been demonstrated in animal studies although not yet in depressed humans.) Newer theories stress the relative amounts of different neurotransmitters rather than the absolute amounts of each one individually. Researchers are also looking at "second messenger systems," activated when neurotransmitters bind themselves to various receptors. These newer theories are highly sophisticated and obviously beyond the scope of this book.

When a person experiences prolonged sadness or grief, the brain's neurotransmitter systems and functioning are thrown off balance. According to the latest research, the neurotransmitters most affected are serotonin, norepinephrine, and possibly dopamine. In **healthy** people the imbalance is corrected; sometimes this takes a few hours, sometimes a few days. In cases of severe grief, like the loss of a close and dear relative, it may take several months.

On the other hand, people who are ill with depression have a chronic imbalance of neurotransmitters and malfunctioning of neurotransmitter systems. This lasts for over two weeks and often much longer. People with a slight imbalance have mild depression. Those with a large imbalance are ill with major (deep) depression.

A similar but reverse imbalance of neurotransmitters could bring on mania, the opposite of depression.

Medicines to treat depression counteract the imbalance and malfunctioning of these brain carriers. Most work by acting on the neurotransmitters serotonin, norepinephrine, and/or dopamine. The way they do this is complicated and not yet fully understood by medical researchers. Newer explanations of why depression occurs and how medicines work are constantly being found and explored.

Some patients ask their doctors to measure the neurotransmitters in their brain and verify that there really is an imbalance and, if so, how much of one. This is pointless and impractical. At present, the experts do not yet understand precisely the biological origin of depression and the way the medicines work. Although, this may seem worrying, there is no need to be concerned. The main thing is that the medicines work.

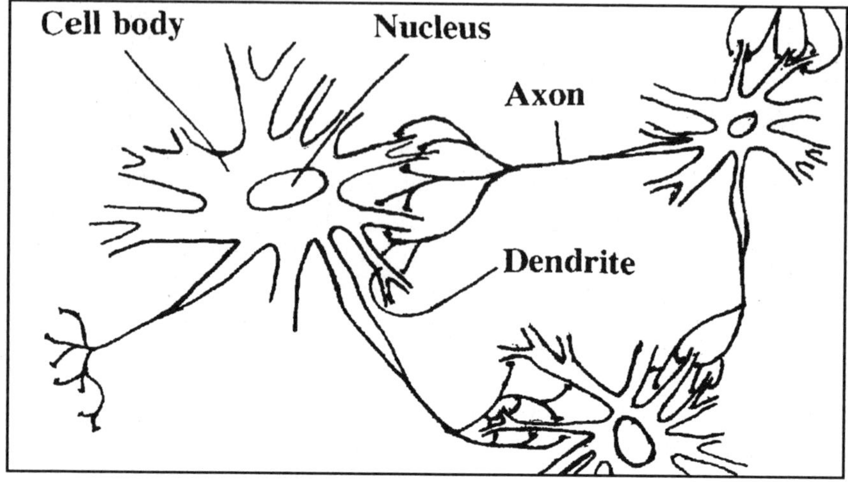

Figure 1. Brain nerve cells

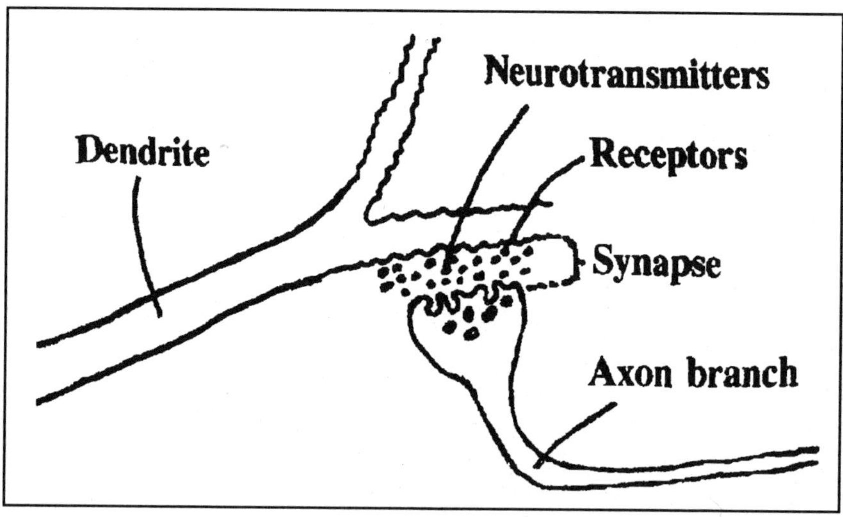

Figure 2. Chemical messengers flowing between brain nerve endings

> *Our creator wisely designed the human body so that we can neither pat ourselves on our own backs nor kick ourselves too easily.*
>
> Anonymous

Chapter 4

205 Reasons to Get Depressed

Depression sometimes comes of itself without any apparent cause. Often, however, it is triggered off by one or a series of upsetting events (even when the underlying cause is a biochemical imbalance in the brain). Life is full of slings and arrows. There are countless reasons why you should feel depressed. Here are 205 of them:

A. Domestic matters

1. Your spouse walks out on you
2. You get divorced
3. You break up with a boyfriend/girlfriend
4. You have an argument with your in-laws
5. You have a bitter custody battle over the children in the courts
6. Your child/children get into a ferocious fight
7. You have an argument with your husband/wife
8. The house is in a big mess
9. The birthday surprise you prepare so carefully turns into a disaster
10. The romantic meal you cook so lovingly gets burned
11. Your baby screams all day and night and you cannot get any sleep
12. Your baby is not developing as fast as you wish
13. You cannot control your toddler who keeps running into mischief
14. Your baby is coming down with strange illnesses
15. All the family is ill, including the children, and you feel exhausted
16. It is vacation time and the children are running wild around the house
17. Your child is neglecting his (her) studies

18. ✓Your child is getting poor academic grades in school
19. Your child is misbehaving at school
20. ✓Your child is mentally disturbed/deficient

21. Your child has a tantrum in front of your friends
22. Your teenager is into a rebellious phase
23. Your teenager hangs out with bad company
24. Your teenager goes out with a boyfriend/girlfriend you dislike
25. Your teenager starts drinking heavily

26. Your teenager starts out on drugs
27. ✓Your teenager always leaves his (her) room in a mess
28. Your teenager dyes his (her) hair a strange color
29. Your teenager plays loud music late at night
30. Your son/daughter marries someone whom you cannot stand

31. ✓You think you look ugly
32. ✓You are disfigured by acne
33. You are going bald
34. You had a hair perm which went all wrong
35. ✓Your clothes no longer fit

36. You have a splitting headache
37. ✓You have come down with a bad cold or the flu
38. You stomach is very upset and you cannot eat
39. You break your leg in accident
40. You have painful arthritis

41. Your landlord doubles the rent
42. You get evicted from your apartment
43. You cannot afford the mortgage payments
44. ✓Your house needs urgent repairs
45. Your builder does shoddy work and charges far too much

46. Your neighbors are unpleasant
47. Your neighbors are putting on loud parties with blaring pop music that lasts until two o'clock in the morning
48. Your neighbor refuses to control his (her) dog who is fierce, barks continually, and frightens the kids
49. Your neighbor lights smelly bonfires on a hot, sultry day
50. Your neighbor's guests block your driveway with their cars

51. You buy an expensive appliance which turns out to be junk
52. The washing machine breaks down for the umpteenth time
53. The heating system fails on a freezing cold day
54. The air conditioning fails on a humid, 100-degree summer day
55. The repair man takes hours to arrive and does a bad job

B. Finance

56. Inflation is on the march
57. Taxes increase
58. ✓You spend more than you earn
59. ✓You get a pay cut or fail to earn a bonus
60. You fall heavily into debt
61. You get sued for $1 million for personal injury because of an accident; legal fees, hours with your attorney, and enormous worry loom ahead
62. The bailiffs come round to your house
63. ✓Your spouse, son or daughter spends heavily on your credit cards without your knowledge
64. Your teenager talks for hours on expensive "900" number telephone calls; you have to foot the bill

> *There is nothing so small that it can't blow itself up out of all proportion.*
>
> Anonymous

C. Work problems

65. ✓You get missed out for promotion
66. ✓You do not get that pay raise
67. Your fellow workers let you down
68. ✓The office "bully" makes your life a misery
69. Your boss is a tyrant
70. ✓You are overloaded with work
71. ✓You have more responsibility than you can take
72. ✓An important deadline approaches which is impossible to meet
73. You are not given enough responsibility
74. Your manager interferes constantly
75. Your manager is incompetent

76. You find your tasks boring
77. Your presentation is a flop
78. You fail to achieve your target
79. The secretary makes a mess of your typing
80. The important meeting is canceled

81. The computer goes down and you have to do everything by hand
82. Irate customers or clients shout at you all day
83. Your manager reprimands you
84. You cannot stand your boss
85. Your subordinates do not pull their weight

86. You work long hours for little pay
87. Your husband/wife wants you to spend more time at home
88. You have too little time in which to relax
89. You are overworked and need a vacation
90. Higher management is uncommunicative; you hardly know what is going on

91. Fear of a recession
92. There is talk of redundancies in the air
93. Your company has just been taken over
94. A comprehensive reorganization is taking place
95. You are let go

96. You are fired for something beyond your control
97. You lose your job as a result of some else's incompetency
98. You are verbally abused
99. You are sexually harassed by your boss
100. You are accused of sexual harassment

101. You face internal discipline
102. You lose your job in disgrace
103. You are self-employed and business is bad
104. A customer has swindled you
105. Your suppliers have let you down

106. It is tax season
107. Your old enemy, the Internal Revenue Service, is after you again with an audit

D. Moving house

108. You are leaving old friends behind
109. You are moving away from your parents, children, brothers, sisters, etc.
110. You dread having to make new friends in an unfamiliar area
111. You are nervous about abandoning old, familiar ways and learning new routines
112. Organizing the move is stressful
113. The removal company breaks some items
114. The removal company loses your favorite sofa
115. Moving house costs much more than you imagined
116. The children are finding it hard to settle down in a new school
117. The cost of living is greater in the new place
118. The weather is colder or wetter

E. Illness and death

119. You are ill with a high temperature, and feel weak and rotten
120. Your spouse and/or children are ill and need looking after
121. Your staff are ill with the flu and you are desperate
122. Treatment is expensive and you do not have enough insurance
123. The doctor is not attentive enough
124. You have to go to bed and miss an event you or your family were looking forward to very much
125. A close member of your family (perhaps your father or mother) is seriously ill
126. You leave your job to nurse that relative
127. Nursing drains the strength from you and you worry a great deal
128. You cannot bear to see him (her) suffer
129. You feel utterly helpless
130. Your standard of living falls because of treatment and nursing costs
131. √The death of a close family member
132. The agony of the last few days
133. √The strain of the funeral

134. Coming to grips with the loss
135. Coping with the grief of a loved one
136. The family squabbles over the will
137. You looked after the dying relative for years but were left hardly anything in the will
138. You are left with a mountain of debt
139. Distributing the dead relative's effects
140. Rebuilding your life after the death of your parent, spouse or child
141. Getting used to life without a dear friend
142. Losing one's favorite pet

F. Information technology and television

143. Getting used to new hi-tech equipment
144. Learning how to use a computer
145. Getting confused by technological complexities which are way above your head
146. Fear of computers "taking over"
147. Losing your job because of computerization
148. Your kids are playing computer games all day instead of doing their homework
149. Too much violence on television
150. Your children are getting "square eyes" watching videos
151. Your bank card gets swallowed up by the automated teller machine
152. The computer is "down" and the automated teller machine refuses to issue you with money; you are stuck without cash
153. Phantom withdrawals from your bank account via the computer
154. Computer fraud frightens you
155. Laser directed missiles fly out of control

G. International affairs

156. Wars between nations
157. Terrorists main and kill hundreds in a huge bomb explosion
158. Global warming, famines and epidemics
159. The threat of a nuclear attack
160. The apparent impotence of the United Nations

H. Accidents and disasters

161. Your car breaks down in the middle of nowhere
162. Getting snarled up in a traffic jam
163. Traffic accidents
164. Dealing with the police after an accident
165. Grappling with insurance claims

166. Dealing with an injury
167. Being incapacitated and off work for months
168. Being a victim of a natural disaster
169. You lose your possessions in a flood
170. Your house gets destroyed by a storm, hurricane, tornado

171. You or your home get struck by lightning
172. An earthquake makes you homeless
173. A friend or relative is injured or lost
174. Putting your life back together after a tragedy

I. Unhappy life experiences

175. Growing up disabled

176. Being abused as a child
177. Growing up without parents or in a one-parent family
178. Intense shyness
179. Being victimized by bullies
180. Difficulty in finding a boyfriend/girlfriend

181. Inability to have children
182. Postmenstrual syndrome pains
183. Hormonal changes
184. Living with a chronic illness or disablement
185. The menopause

186. The mid-life crisis
187. Adjusting to retirement and growing old
188. Your children leave home
189. Losing one's physical strength and vitality
190. Living in a retirement home

191. Fear of senility
192. Living through a terminal illness
193. Facing death

J. Miscellaneous

194. The weather: cold, rain, fog, heat, storms, snow, etc.
195. Politics

196. The Republicans/Democrats win the election
197. Prolonged and excessive stress
198. The side effect of powerful medications
199. A hangover after drinking too much alcohol
200. Drug and substance abuse

201. Hearing sad music
202. Lowering of spirits caused by certain illnesses
203. Brain damage as the result of an accident or a stroke
204. No apparent cause; sadness just comes out of the blue
205. Spending holidays (e.g., Thanksgiving and Christmas) alone or in the company of relatives you dislike but are expected to meet

> *Life can be understood by looking backward, but it must be lived by looking forward.*
>
> Sören Aabye Kierkegaard (1813–1855)

Chapter 5

Symptoms of Depression

The symptoms of depression can be divided roughly into three classes: physical, emotional and other.

Physical symptoms of depression

1. **Sleep disturbances.** Do you find it difficult to fall asleep at night? Do you wake up in the middle of the night and find it hard to fall asleep again? Do you feel so tired during the day that you fall asleep at work? Alternatively, do you constantly oversleep?

2. **Appetite and bowel disturbances.** Overeating **or** undereating. Frequent diarrhea or constipation.

3. **Loss of sex drive.** Even when you love your spouse or partner and **want** to have sex.

4. **Fatigue and decreased energy.** Do you feel constantly exhausted? Do you often feel as though you are dragging yourself through the day? Do you feel unrefreshed after a sleep?

5. **Panic attacks.** Characterized by some or all of the following: rapid heart beat, shortness of breath, faintness, dizziness, chest pains, tingling, a sense of impending danger and doom (without knowing what), and an intense fear of losing control or going crazy. Sometimes triggered by a stressful event or memory; sometimes comes by itself out of the blue.

> *Nothing in life is to be feared; it is only to be understood.*
>
> Marie Curie (1867–1934)

Emotional symptoms of depression

1. **Sadness and despair.** Have you, for more than two weeks or so, felt sad, gloomy, empty, disappointed, and "blue"? Do you feel heartache and/or heaviness in the pit of the stomach? Do you often cry or feel like crying? Feeling sadness and despair is normal for short periods, but not for as long as two weeks at a time.

2. **Anhedonia.** Inability to experience pleasure. No zest for life. Do activities you used to enjoy no longer interest you?

3. **Low self-esteem.** Do you feel worthless and inadequate? Do you lack confidence? Do you sometimes even hate yourself? Do you often tell yourself: "I'm no good" or "I'm useless" or "I can't do it" or "I never do anything right"?

   Do you feel you need to please everybody, even people who take advantage of or mistreat you? Do you often feel inferior to others (even when this is not true)? Do you usually defer to other people's opinions and guidance? Do you find it difficult to persuade others of your own ideas and opinions?

4. **Apathy.** Poor motivation. Loss of interest in life. Social withdrawal. Do you often tell yourself: "What's the point? I don't feel like going out and being with others." Do you find it hard to arouse interest in yourself to do something you used to love doing in the past?

   Failure to engage in social and recreational activities eventually leads to life becoming less and less meaningful. In other words, a vicious circle develops leading to more pronounced depression. This is one of the worst aspects of depression: an illness which feeds upon itself.

5. **Interpersonal problems.** Difficulty in having a healthy, satisfying relationship with other people. Are you extremely sensitive to criticism and rejection? Do you feel uncomfortable or inadequate around other people? Do you experience frequent and intense feelings of loneliness?

   Do you find it difficult to be assertive? Are you often taken advantage of by other people? Do you find it hard to say no?

Do you sometimes become unreasonably irritable or angry at other people, even your best friends? Have you lost friends because of this?

6. **Guilt feelings.** Feeling excessively remorseful, regretful, or bad about yourself. This is another of the vicious things about depression: sometimes the guilt feelings are so strong that you feel very guilty about facing up to the possibility of having depression and too ashamed to tell anyone about it. Therefore, you do not seek help and you spoil your chances of a quick recovery.

©ASHLEIGH BRILLIANT 1983.
POT-SHOTS NO. 2995.
IF I DID ANYTHING WRONG, I'M SORRY—
Ashleigh Brilliant
IF I DID ANYTHING RIGHT, I'M PLEASANTLY SURPRISED.

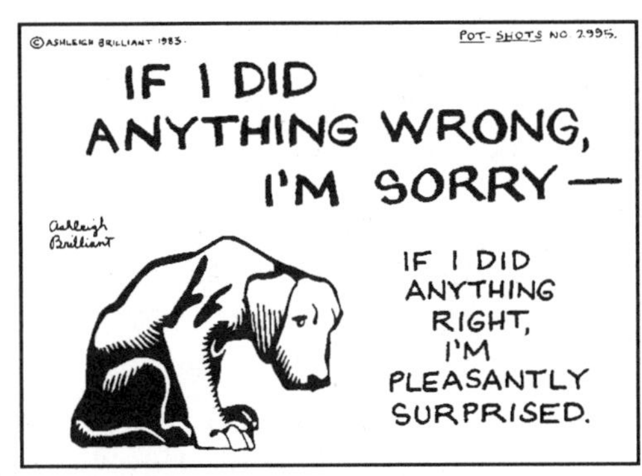

7. **Negative thinking.** Psychiatrists call this "cognitive distortion." Do you tend to see things in a negative, pessimistic way? This is another way in which depressive illness deepens and prolongs itself.

8. **Suicidal thoughts.** Do you feel like ending your life or "disappearing" from the world? Do you hope you will be run over by a truck or a train? Is life not worth living anymore? Thoughts like these are not natural in a healthy person; they reflect a curable illness. You probably will not believe this if you often have suicidal thoughts, but it is true.

Treatment is warranted even if you have not actually attempted suicide. If you have, then your depression is extremely deep. Gather your strength and seek help immediately!

> *The difficulties of life are intended to make us better, not bitter.*
> Anonymous

Other symptoms of depression

1. **Poor concentration.** Difficulty in understanding what is being said or going on around. Do you even sometimes wonder whether you are losing your mind? Or whether you are becoming stupid?

2. **Poor recent memory.** Forgetfulness. Is it hard to memorize information? Do you forget things you used to be able to remember easily? Again, you may wonder whether you are losing your mind.

3. **Hypochondria.** Excessive concern with your health. Believing you may be suffering from a dire illness. Are you afraid you may have cancer? A heart attack? Alzheimer's disease? Early onset of senility?

   Do you feel aches and pains symptomatic of these illnesses? You may. Throbbing pains across the chest. Severe headaches. Pains in the bowels. Nausea. Difficulty in focusing the mind. Obsession with thoughts you cannot get your mind away from. Perhaps a combination of all of these. A very painful combination. However, your doctor examines you and cannot find anything wrong.

   The pain is real enough. The good news is that you do not have any of these deadly illnesses. It is probably this sinister enemy, depression, which is extremely adept at mimicking these illnesses. With treatment, these mysterious and frightening pains will gradually disappear. At this point in time, you may not believe it; but it is true.

4. **Drug and/or alcohol abuse.** What do many people do to lift their spirits, to relieve the "doom and gloom"? Have a drink, of course. What happens when they have depression and constantly feel miserable? Have lots of drinks. Get drunk. Wake up with hangovers. Have more drinks. And get addicted. Is this you or someone you know?

   A similar story applies to frequent drug users.

It is reckoned that a third to a half of drug and alcohol abusers are addicted only because they are suffering from depression. Cure lies through treating the depression.

5. **Excessive emotional sensitivity** (including anger and irritability). Do you often feel an intense, overwhelming surge of emotion in response to minor happenings which hardly affect other people? For example, anger and tearfulness?

6. **Pronounced mood swings.** Does your mood frequently change from sad to very sad and back again? Or from sad to very happy (euphoria) and vice versa? Is your mood taking control of your life, and making it feel unbearable as a result?

7. **Family history** of depression, manic-depression, suicide, eating disorders, or alcoholism. (This not strictly speaking a "symptom" but a predisposing factor.) Do you have a close relative who has or has had depression? Depression tends to run in families which means that relatives are more vulnerable to the illness.

A person does not need to exhibit **all** the above symptoms in order to have depression. Doctors will diagnose this illness when someone has the majority of these symptoms. They may refer to the Diagnostic and Statistics Manual (DSM) IV, published by the American Psychiatric Association (APA), for guidance. This manual defines various levels of severity for depression and other mind disorders.

Some people with depression, especially hypochondriacs and drug abusers, are convinced that they are not ill with depression at all. They put down their symptoms to other causes. Their depression is said to be "masked." Successful treatment depends on persuading them that they really have depression, after all.

> *The way I look at it, if you want the rainbow, you gotta put up with the rain.*
>
> Dolly Parton

Chapter 6

Why Most Sufferers are not Diagnosed, or Wrongly Diagnosed, or Badly Treated

Depression is an illness most people associate with feeling low, being unable to get out of bed in the morning and, ultimately, committing suicide.

Actually, it is more widespread in its mild form than most people imagine. Research by leading institutions in Britain and America shows that one in twenty people have it without knowing it. This is because it often masquerades as other illnesses. The symptoms are not as dramatic as those above but are devastating all the same. Frequent headaches, nausea, tiredness, appetite problems, "nerves," and the like.

© ASHLEIGH BRILLIANT 1983
POT-SHOTS NO. 3119
I'VE ACCUMULATED ENOUGH TO BE THE ENVY OF ALL MY FRIENDS,
IF I HAD ANY FRIENDS.
Ashleigh Brilliant

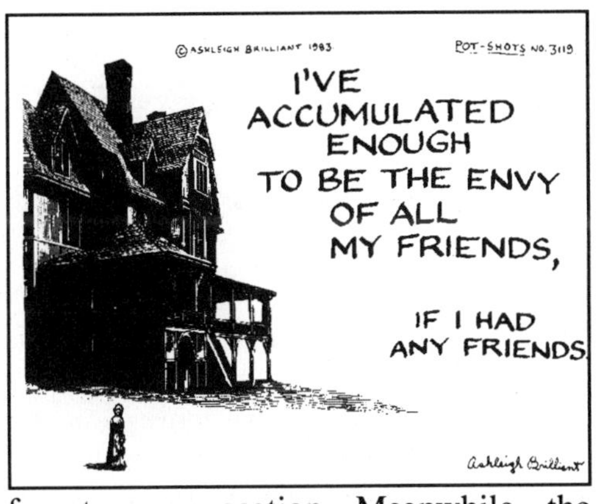

What often happens is that people affected take aspirins, stomach settlers, vitamins, tranquilizers, etc. on an ongoing basis. If the symptoms continue long enough, they might go to their family doctors. And what might the doctors do? Prescribe more medicines to treat the symptoms they are told about. Maybe they will recommend a period of rest or a vacation. Meanwhile, the depression remains untreated and the symptoms return.

Unfortunately, many doctors are not trained well enough to delve down deeper and recognize depression. And many of those that do correctly diagnose the illness prescribe insufficient or the wrong type of medicine so the patients do not make a good recovery. It is estimated that only one in three doctors properly diagnose and treat the illness.

Another serious problem is that the illness makes people feel lethargic, insecure, guilty and ashamed of themselves. Some may feel too guilty and ashamed to admit their feelings to their doctor. Others may feel too lethargic to make the visit and give up. Yet others may react by putting on an act of well-being and cheerfulness; they think it would be weak-spirited to do otherwise.

The end result is that their doctor cannot find out that they are ill. Therefore, they cannot get treated. Many remain ill and suffer for a long time. That is one of the worst aspects of depression; it is a horribly self-defeating illness.

In the saddest cases, people receive treatment only on becoming so ill that they make a suicide attempt, or lose their job, or something equally horrendous happens in their life. It is a terrible tragedy that they have to go to such extreme pain and suffering before they can recover.

The good news is that there are now so many treatments available, that doctors can treat over 95 in 100 cases of depression successfully. Dreary pain and seemingly endless suffering, features of this illness, can be put behind for most people.

INTERESTING FACTS

Did you know that depression is more common than most people think? For example:

1. Approximately 10% of the population (estimated) are ill without their realizing.
2. Only one in three doctors properly diagnose and treat depression.
3. Recent advances mean a 95+% success rate when the illness is properly treated.
4. The tragedy of the illness lies in its nature; sufferers do not feel like seeking help, and easily give up trying.

A problem well stated is a problem half solved.

Anonymous

PART TWO:

MEDICAL TREATMENT

Chapter 7

How to Avoid Spending a Fortune

No one should condemn themselves to continual sadness by putting on a brave face and doing nothing. The most sensible thing to do is find a treatment that makes one better. There are two main approaches: psychotherapy and medicine. One of these or both is appropriate, depending on the type of depression.

Treatment usually takes place over a long time period and, therefore, it can be expensive. Unfortunately, health insurance plans put strict limits on mental health treatment these days. This may put off a lot of people. (Although, it is unfair and discriminatory, we will have to live with this fact until the insurance companies have a change of heart.)

©ASHLEIGH BRILLIANT 1983.
POT-SHOTS NO. 2844.
WITH PSYCHIATRIC HELP SO EXPENSIVE AND TIME-CONSUMING, I CAN'T AFFORD TO BE MORE THAN SLIGHTLY UNHAPPY.

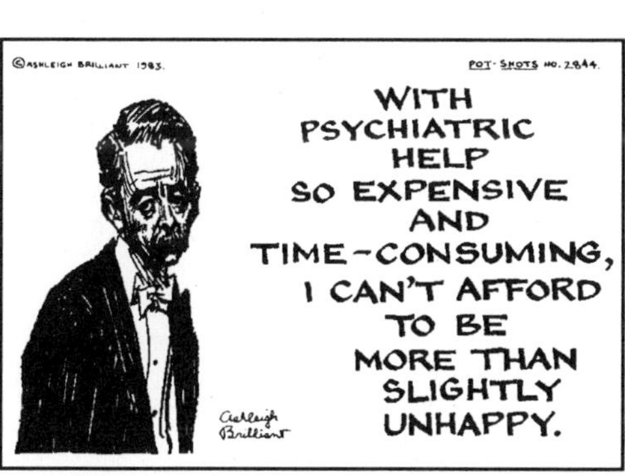

The good news is that it does not have to be expensive with the right approach. This section explains what you can do to make sure you get all the treatment you need without going bankrupt.

At this point the author has to point out a sad and unpleasant fact which he is sure that the medical profession will be very reluctant to admit. While most psychiatrists and psychotherapists undoubtedly do their very professional best, there are a number of unscrupulous individuals around who take advantage of depressed people by giving them prolonged and/or unnecessary treatment at great cost.

Without doubt, the medical profession would protest by exclaiming that a patient can easily switch to another doctor or make a complaint to the appropriate authority. However, this is easy to do in theory but difficult, sometimes impossible, in practice because of the very nature of the illness. Depression is characterized by a lack of confidence, weak spiritedness, low energy, poor concentration, suggestibility, etc. How can depressed people be expected to be fully assertive?

This section explains what you can do to avoid falling into this unpleasant trap.

Let no one suppose that the words doctor and patient can disguise from the parties that they are employer and employee.

George Bernard Shaw (1856–1950)

Chapter 8

When to Seek Professional Help

The exact time to seek professional help is usually a personal decision, depending on the depth and duration of your symptoms and the amount of your discomfort. The exception, of course, is in an emergency situation when immediate action is required.

Generally speaking, you should seek an evaluation if you experience feelings, thoughts or actions like the following:

1. An emotional or mental difficulty makes you change some important aspect of your life. Examples:
(a) You no longer go out with friends because your mind keeps returning to a problem you just can't seem to resolve.
(b) You find yourself withdrawing from family or friends because you're feeling inexplicably angry at them.
(c) You're taking sick days at work because when you get there you can't seem to concentrate.
(d) You have decided not to continue school because you can't take the social pressure or the competition.
(e) You've stopped driving your car because sometimes you get terribly panicky.

2. You feel generally displeased with yourself. Examples:
✓(a) You hate yourself because you think you are fat or ugly.
✓(b) You feel you should be doing better than you are in various aspects of your life but for some reason you're not.
(c) You feel lonely and isolated and you don't know why you can't seem to connect to others.
(d) You feel continuously guilty or bad about some of your thoughts, feelings, or actions toward others.
✓(e) You can't assert your feelings or desires.
✓(f) You wish you weren't so nervous all the time.

3. You feel generally displeased with life or with others. Examples:
(a) People you meet always seem to have things better than you do.
✓(b) The activities you have always enjoyed enormously no longer seem fun.
(c) Life seems to have no purpose or point to it, and you don't see much hope that it ever will.
(d) You feel out of touch with those around you or with life in general.
✓(e) People are always blaming you for things that you believe are their fault.
✓(f) You believe that your life is too stressful and you are losing your ability to cope.
(g) You feel your habits or actions are out of control.
(h) You are angry at your doctor, who keeps telling you that your physical symptoms have no organic basis.

> *Many people admire a good loser—as long as it's somebody else.*
> Anonymous

4. You are unhappy about your relationships. Examples:
✓(a) You always seem to get into relationships with people who harm or take advantage of you.
(b) You can't seem to grow really close to or become intimate with others.
✓(c) You and your partner cannot establish a satisfying relationship, sexually or otherwise.
(d) You are never happy for long in a relationship.
✓(e) You worry so much all the time or are so moody that nobody seems to want to put up with you.

5. You have a hunch that your drinking or drug use is getting out of control. Examples:
(a) You habitually drink early in the morning.
(b) You drive a car while you are high on drugs.
(c) You ask your family doctor for more and more sleeping pills or tranquilizers.
(d) People in your life are telling you that you have a drinking or drug problem, and you find yourself reacting angrily at them.

What should you do if you are concerned for the welfare of a friend or close relative who is not behaving like his (her) normal, happy self? Certain types of behavior might cause you to become concerned for someone who is close to you. Where feasible, it is best for the troubled person to initiate treatment personally. It can be difficult, however, to convince a reluctant individual to seek mental health assistance. You may wish to arrange for a consultation in which you discuss the problem with a professional yourself and clarify whether you have grounds for your concerns.

©ASHLEIGH BRILLIANT 1983.
POT-SHOTS NO 3006.
Ashleigh Brilliant
IT'S NOT YOU I'M ANGRY AT ~
I'M ANGRY AT MYSELF, FOR LETTING YOU UPSET ME.

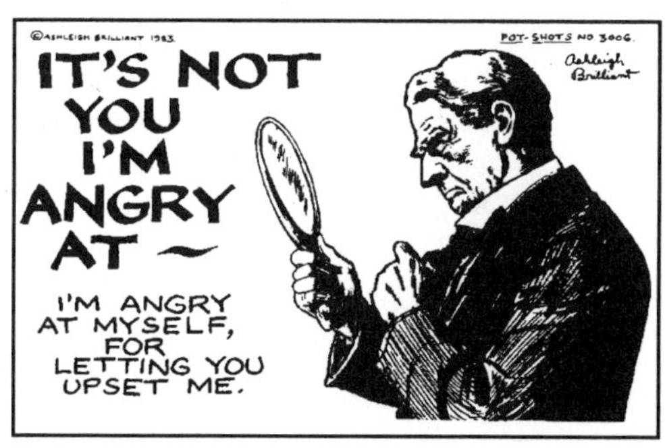

In any case, if the demeanor or behavior of someone close to you causes you concern, always talk to him (her) about it first. Support, attention from others, and the chance to air their worries can provide great comfort and relief for people who are troubled. In the case of children or relatives whom you believe are mentally incompetent, you may wish to arrange for the evaluation personally. Following now are examples of behaviors in others that may alert you to their need for help:

1. The person reacts to events in disproportionate ways. Examples:
   (a) Your spouse or child repeatedly loses his (her) temper over trivial events.
   (b) Your child's bitterness over an "unfair" grade seems to increase rather than ebb as the weeks pass.
   (c) Your relative believes that your concern for him (her) means, "You're out to get me."

2. The person has had a major mood or behavior change. Examples:
   (a) Your spouse has lost interest in talking about the day's events and prefers to sit alone and brood every evening.
   (b) Your father hasn't recovered from the death of your mother three years ago and seems to be getting even sadder day by day.
   (c) Your normally happy-go-lucky daughter has not smiled in weeks and has begun to do poorly in school after having performed well in the past.

(d) A family member has become extremely forgetful and confused.
(e) Since the birth of your child, your wife has been weeping all the time and claiming she's not a good mother.
(f) Your teenage son, a longtime fan of rock music, has started giving away all his favorite recordings.
(g) A relative who always used to dress neatly has begun to go to work grossly unkempt.
(h) You've begun to notice that every time your spouse is about to leave the house, he (she) must return to the kitchen repeatedly to check that the stove is turned off.
(i) A family member suddenly has become fearful of situations that he (she) tolerated in the past.
(j) Your apparently healthy relative has been visiting one doctor after another searching for the physician who will finally diagnose and treat some mysterious illness.
(k) Your child, spouse, or relative has periods in which he (she) seems too happy, overly optimistic, and excessively energetic, with strangely little need for sleep.
(l) The person has begun acting in extremely risky ways while denying that his (her) behavior is dangerous.

An emergency situation is at hand if a person is suicidal or represents a physical danger to himself (herself). Examples:

1. Suicidal behavior. Anything from minor wrist-cutting to severe body mutilation or dangerous overdoses of drugs requires immediate action. Help should be sought at the hospital emergency room, or by telephoning the local suicide hot-line.

2. Suicidal statements. The same should be done in the case of a person who announces a wish to be dead if he (she) has been depressed for a considerable time, or has been abusing drugs or drink. However, no action need be taken when someone is just momentarily depressed over an upsetting incident and is merely expressing frustration.

> *It's not that I'm afraid to die; I just don't want to be there when it happens.*
>
> Woody Allen (1935–)

Chapter 9

The Different Kinds of Mental Health Professionals

Mental health professionals are experienced in one or more of the following fields: psychiatry, psychology, social work, psychiatric nursing, and counseling. Only those accredited by a reputable, professional organization should be used. This is because it is an unfortunate fact that nowadays anyone in the United States can set themselves up as a "psychotherapist," "psychoanalyst," "counselor," etc. without any training or qualifications whatsoever! Impressive though they sound, these terms have no legal meaning and there is no requirement for licensing.

U.S. MENTAL HEALTH PROFESSIONALS

Psychiatrists	41,000
Psychologists	65,000
Social workers	81,000
Psychiatric nurses	33,000
Mental health counselors (licensed)	46,000
TOTAL (approximate numbers)	**266,000**

1. **Psychiatrists.** These are highly specialized medical doctors licensed by the state in which they practice. The most expensive of the mental health professionals, they are the only ones entitled to prescribe drugs and admit patients to hospital.

   Psychiatrists are required to go through long and extensive training. First they have to complete four years in medical school, then one year of internship, and finally three years residency. They are trained in neurology, clinical medical care, and child, adolescent and geriatric psychiatry. They learn about inpatient, outpatient and emergency treatment, gaining intensive, practical experience in a wide range of psychiatric disorders.

   After graduation, most psychiatrists seek certification from the American Board of Psychiatry and Neurology (ABPN). In order to do this, they must pass written and oral examinations. Then they practice either general psychiatry or specialize in areas such as child psychiatry or substance abuse treatment.

   Besides being able to prescribe medications, psychiatrists can diagnose and evaluate any underlying organic disease, and coordinate the treatment with other medical specialists. (Other mental health professionals are not in a position to do this.) Therefore, they are well placed to treat serious mental illnesses such as severe depression for which medication is usually required.

   Psychiatrists are also trained in psychotherapy and are entitled to practice in it. However, they may not be as proficient as psychologists since they are more likely to pursue specialized training in other areas such as psychopharmacology (described below). For this reason, it may be more desirable to see a psychiatrist for medication and a psychologist for psychotherapy. Moreover, psychologists usually charge much less. (Psychotherapy is very time consuming.)

   Psychopharmacologists are psychiatrists who specialize in the therapeutic use of medications.

A list of psychiatrists with qualifications and experience can be obtained from a directory published by the American Psychiatric Association (APA) at 1400 K Street, NW, Washington, DC 20005 (tel. 202-682-6000). Most psychiatrists belong to this organization. The directory can be found in the local library. Unfortunately, the list is in alphabetical order of names which is not helpful for finding the best psychiatrist in the local area quickly.

Better still is the annual "Directory of Certified Psychiatrists" published by the American Board of Medical Specialties (ABMS) at 1007 Church Street, Suite 404, IL 60201 Evanston, (tel. 708-491-9091), in collaboration with the American Board of Psychiatry and Neurology. This directory, which can also be found in large public libraries, contains both a list of psychiatrists in the order of city and state, and also a list of qualifications and experience in alphabetical order of names.

2. **Psychologists.** Delving into a person's personality and behavior, a psychologist tries to understand the factors behind his (her) emotional problems. By means of psychotherapy, the psychologist helps the patient identify problem areas and build up a healthier and more robust emotional outlook.

Besides studying for a doctorate in clinical psychology and passing a state licensing examination, psychologists must undergo practical training for at least one year followed by one year of supervised part-time practice. Training includes study of general psychology, personality theory, psychodynamics, and therapeutic techniques.

> *To profit from good advice requires as much wisdom as to give it.*
> Anonymous

Many psychologists work in collaboration with psychiatrists. In this arrangement, the psychologist concentrates on therapy and psychological assessment while the psychiatrist provides medications and general medical care. Some psychologists specialize, e.g., in children's problems or marital guidance.

A list of psychologists can be obtained from a directory published by the American Psychological Association, located at 750 First Street, NE, Washington, DC 20002 (tel. 202-336-5500). Most psychologists belong to this organization. The directory is obtainable at large public libraries. Check that the psychologist has been awarded a diploma of excellence from the American Board of Professional Psychology. This diploma is given only after five years of post-doctoral experience and rigorous examinations.

An alternative list of state certified or licensed psychologists can be obtained from a register kept by the National Register of Health Service Providers in Psychology, 1120 G Street, NW, Suite 330, Washington, DC 20005 (tel. 202-783-7663). However, inclusion in the register does not guarantee extensive practical experience in psychotherapy.

3. **Social workers.** Psychiatric social workers can also provide psychotherapy and often work in collaboration with psychiatrists. Most have a master's degree in social work which includes two years of classroom instruction and at least nine hundred hours of supervised clinical practice. A social worker's expertise may be just as good as a psychologist's.

A list of social workers can be obtained from registers kept by two professional organizations: (a) the National Association of Social Workers, Inc. (NASW) (Register of Clinical Social Workers) at 750 First Street, NE, Suite 700, Washington, DC 20002 (tel. 800-638-8799 or 202-408-8600) and (b) the American Board of Examiners in Clinical Social Work at 3 Mill Road, Suite 306, Wilmington, DE 19806 (tel. 302-739-4522). Both hold details of social workers who apply and satisfy certain formal criteria.

Advice is like snow; the softer it falls, the longer it dwells upon, and the deeper it sinks into, the mind.

Samuel Taylor Coleridge (1772–1834)

4. **Psychiatric nurses.** Besides applying general nursing skills, these professionals closely monitor and document the progress of their patients in hospital, and coordinate treatment with psychiatrists and other mental health professionals. They receive specialized training, both theoretical and practical, in mental health care. This includes physical and emotional aspects, methods of psychotherapy, and various types of medications with their actions and side effects. Widespread and thorough practical experience is obtained and some practitioners study up to a master's degree.

   A list of certified psychiatric nurses can be obtained from the American Nurses Association at 600 Maryland Avenue, SW, Suite 100, Washington, DC 20024 (tel. 202-554-4444). Certification is awarded only after a minimum of two years postgraduate practice (including one hundred hours of supervised work) and passing a qualifying examination.

5. **Mental health counselors.** Anyone can call himself (herself) by this title so credentials must be checked carefully. A counselor should at least be certified by the National Academy of Certified Clinical Mental Health Counselors which is an arm of the American Mental Health Counselors Association (AMHCA) at 5999 Stevenson Avenue, Alexandria, VA 22304 (tel. 703-823-9800, ext. 383).

   The title of Certified Clinical Mental Health Counselor is granted after obtaining a master's degree in mental health counseling, spending three thousand hours in supervised, postgraduate practical work, and passing a national qualifying examination. About only one in forty members of the AMHCA have this title.

   A large group of counselors (called pastoral counselors) are members of the clergy. Many are very skilled in psychotherapy and sorting out personal problems. Their services are likely to be much cheaper than those of the other professionals which is a big plus. One can have the confidence that the clergyman (or clergywoman) is working from the heart, and is not out to spend lots of time in therapy trying to make as much money as possible.

A pastoral counselor can become certified by the American Association of Pastoral Counselors at 9504A Lee Highway, Fairfax, VA 22031 (tel. 703-385-6967). Certification is granted after a three-year graduate program in divinity studies, and a master's degree or doctorate theology program that includes clinical training in crisis intervention. However, certification is not required by law to practice as a pastoral counselor.

Other mental health counselors may call themselves marriage and family therapists, sex therapists, substance abuse counselors, etc. At present, there is no national certification program. Therefore, these practitioners should be chosen with great care. Organizations which can assist are the following:

(a) the American Family Therapy Association at 2020 Pennsylvania Avenue, NW, Suite 273, Washington, DC 20006 (tel. 202-994-2776)

(b) the American Association of Sex Educators, Counselors and Therapists at 435 North Michigan Avenue, Suite 1717, Chicago, IL 60611 (tel. 312-644-0828)

(c) the National Association of Alcohol and Drug Counselors at 1911 North Fort Myer Drive, Suite 900, Arlington, VA 22209 (tel. 703-741-7686)

> *Everyone's allowed an occasional failure—except the skydiver, of course.*
>
> Anonymous

Chapter 10

Methods of Treatment: An Overview

There are two main approaches to healing mental disorders, including depression. The first is taking medications prescribed by a doctor. The second is talking over problems, emotions and feelings with a trained professional; this is called psychotherapy.

Psychotherapy can be used by itself or in conjunction with medication. When used by itself, it is most effective for people with mild to moderate depression. However, when the depression is severe, the patient usually loses the motivation and attention necessary in order to absorb the treatment efficiently. In such a case, the best approach is to first take medication. Once the depression becomes moderate or mild, psychotherapy can then play an important role.

Medications can also be very effective in treating mild or moderate depression without psychotherapy. In general, however, the best results come from a combination of both these approaches to treatment.

A course of psychotherapy may last longer and cost significantly more than a course of medication. Psychotherapy typically takes months (sometimes years) to work, whereas medications are usually effective in a matter of weeks. The former also requires more time spent with the mental health practitioner. This translates into higher medical charges. Therefore, when time and cost are important factors, it generally makes more sense to try out medications first and then psychotherapies, rather than the other way around.

In the minority of cases when a course of treatment fails to work, you may need to switch over to a different course of treatment. While you can find out if a prescribed medication does not work after only about eight weeks, it can take you a few months or possibly more than a year to find out the same about a certain type of psychotherapy.

If you fall into this category, it also may make better sense to spend a few months trying out a couple of medications first and then psychotherapy, rather than spend several years experimenting with different types of therapy first and then medications.

In some people depression tends to be recurrent but of limited duration, lasting six to twelve months even when untreated. Medications and psychotherapy can hasten the recovery and prevent further episodes. At the same time, it is worth being alert to the possibility of recovery happening spontaneously and not on account of the treatment.

It must be emphasized that precise cost benefit analysis of psychotherapy versus medication, including the assessment of risks, is very complicated. Therefore, the above suggestions should only be taken as guide. You are recommended to discuss your individual case thoroughly and carefully with your mental health practitioner before coming to a decision on the best approach to treatment.

Other specialized treatments for depression are electroconvulsive therapy (ECT), phototherapy, biofeedback, nutritional healing, and various drug-free remedies. These are described in more detail in later chapters.

I've developed a new philosophy: I only dread one day at a time.
Charles Schultz (1922–)

Chapter 11

Approaches in Psychotherapy

The most important thing is to have a good rapport with the therapist. He (she) should provide emotional support and reduce psychological pain and distress. Make sure that he (she) describes up front the psychotherapeutic technique(s) to be used, what that translates to in terms of time and money, and the expected results and benefits. If the therapist cannot or will not, it may be a sign that he (she) is either incompetent or is out to have a long, drawn-out series of sessions with you, using you as a source of income. In either case, you would be advised to look for a different therapist.

Ideally, the therapist will produce a program of action with specific goals and time scales. Use it to review your progress and assess the effectiveness of the treatment.

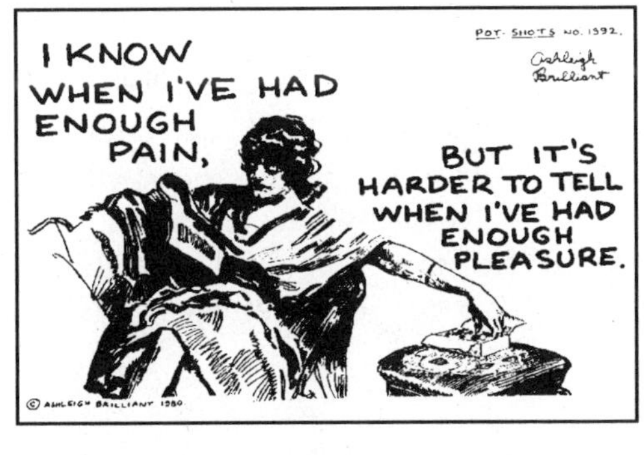

Several therapeutic techniques have been used successfully in treating depression. Your therapist may use a mixture of all of them with a bit of "Dear Abby" type of advice thrown in for good measure. (Some call this approach "supportive" therapy.) The U.S. Department of Health and Human Services (Agency for Health Care Policy and Research) guidelines list three types of therapy which have been shown to be useful in treating mild to moderate depression with an effectiveness equal to that of medications: cognitive-behavior therapy, interpersonal therapy, and behavior therapy. These and other types of therapy are now described.

1. Behavior therapy. Through discussion the patient works out where specific behaviors are inappropriate or undesirable. For example, taking a long time to get out of bed in the morning, constantly arriving late at work, and bursting into tears when even mildly criticized. The idea is that all behaviors are learned and that what is learned can be "unlearned" and/or "relearned." This usually involves an active effort on the part of the therapist and patient, including homework assignments and the like. With constant practice, inappropriate behaviors are modified and undesirable behaviors eliminated. Overall performance and satisfaction in life starts to improve and the depression lifts.

   Behavior therapy is designed to be of a short-term nature, lasting perhaps 10 to 20 sessions over several months.

2. Cognitive-behavior therapy. This is based on the idea that people's behavior and feelings are influenced by the way they think about themselves and the world. For example, an employee who is convinced that all his (her) work is of low quality and that he (she) is unappreciated might perform poorly, resulting in failure to achieve promotion, discouragement, and depression.

   The therapist works with the patient to identify and list problematic thoughts and behaviors, and discover what stimulates them. As with behavior therapy, the patient consciously attempts, with constant practice, to "unlearn" or "relearn" the maladapted thinking in order to produce constructive thoughts, realistic attitudes, and productive behaviors.

   This therapy is also designed to be of a short-term nature, lasting perhaps 10 to 20 sessions over several months.

> *A word of encouragement during failure is worth more than a whole book praise after success.*
>
> Anonymous

3. Interpersonal therapy. The idea behind this therapy is that disturbed social relationships cause depressive symptoms which in turn exacerbate these disturbed relationships and deepen the depression. Treatment focuses on the patient's current interpersonal problems within the framework of one of four areas: grief, interpersonal role disputes, role transitions, or interpersonal deficits.

Grief is bereavement following the death of a loved one, e.g., a spouse. The therapist gradually helps the patient to find new activities and relationships to compensate for the loss.

Interpersonal role disputes are conflicts with a significant other, such as a spouse, family member, fellow worker, or close friend. With the aid of the therapist, the patient considers options to resolve the dispute or replace the relationship with better alternatives.

Role transitions occur on changes in life status. Examples are children leaving home, a new career, promotion, retirement, diagnosis of a severe medical illness, and loss of a treasured ideal. The patient is helped to deal with the changes by recognizing the positive and negative aspects of the new and old roles, and coming to terms with them.

Interpersonal deficits are a consequence of poor social skills, including the ability to initiate and sustain relationships. With the assistance of the therapist, the patient identifies the skills that are lacking and the actions necessary to build them up.

Treatment ends with the patient recognizing and consolidating therapeutic gains and developing ways to identify and counter any future depressive symptoms. The whole process is also relatively short, say, some 15 sessions over a three to four month period.

Interpersonal therapy has also been found to be as effective for treating major depression as some medications.

4. Psychodynamic therapy. Here the therapist investigates with the patient to discover the source of current but unconscious feelings and emotions, and analyzes them in depth. It involves going through the history of when they began and when they developed. Defenses against these feelings and emotions are examined. Developed gradually over time, these defenses are individual to the patient, influenced by temperament as well as environment. It is hoped that, through this process, the patient will understand and comes to grips with his (her) feelings and emotions, and develop more mature and appropriate styles of reacting to situations in life. In this way the depression will lift.

There are three categories of psychodynamic therapy. Psychoanalysis, the original form, is lengthy, intensive, and expensive. Treatment may go on for three to five years at three to five sessions per week. Patients are encouraged to "free associate" (say whatever comes to mind) and discuss their dreams. The psychoanalyst helps the patient to interpret his (her) thoughts, feelings, and fantasies without interference.

Psychoanalytic therapy, a modified form of psychoanalysis, is less intensive and time-consuming. Meetings between patient and therapist may take place one to three times per week for a period of one to five years. Although the patient is still encouraged to express whatever comes to mind, the therapist takes a more active role.

Brief dynamic therapy, a major innovation in psychodynamic therapy, focuses on specific problems and goals. Treatment is limited to usually no more than 25 sessions.

> *Beware the expert: a person who can take something you already know and make it sound confusing.*
>
> Anonymous

5. Family therapy. This is a particularly effective treatment for depression related to problems within the family, e.g., strife between parents and children, and difficulties in marriage. The family is viewed as an interdependent unit, with each member playing a role in maintaining its stability. A depressed child, for example, may sink into depression rather than confront a dominating, overbearing brother or sister. By examining the family structure, communication, and styles of interaction, the therapist helps its members modify their roles and behavior in order to find a healthier, more satisfactory form of stability.

   Family therapy focuses on problems and is usually of short duration. As a result, the family may decide to set new limits for the children; establish firmer boundaries between the roles each generation plays; understand and accept individual differences; and learn new ways to communicate, interact, and express feelings.

   Parents, children, and grandparents comprise the main members of the family unit. On occasion, this may be extended to include stepfamilies and individuals who are unrelated but very involved, e.g., close friends.

   Marital therapy is an offshoot of family therapy which specializes on committed couples. It is very suitable where the depression of a husband or wife is clearly linked to problems within the marriage.

6. Group therapy. Most psychotherapy takes place between only the patient and the therapist. This is called individual psychotherapy. Another successful form, called group therapy, takes place between a group of patients and the therapist at the same time. Sometimes the patients all have similar emotional conditions and circumstances, e.g., depressed adolescents. At other times, they have a mixture of emotional problems, ages, sexes, socioeconomic status, etc.

   Most group therapists base their treatment on interpersonal therapy. Other specialized approaches have names such as: confrontational, repressive/inspirational, time-extended, psychodrama, transactional analysis, structured experiences, and special population group therapy.

The aim of this kind of therapy is to use the social interaction between the members of the group to bring about individual improvements in personality and behavior. There is no need to delve into the problems of each member's current circumstances and past life since they will inevitably be brought up within the group.

Group therapy has many other advantages. Most emotional problems involve relationships and social skills with other people. Therefore, group therapy is a most practical way to make improvements in these areas. It is very supportive knowing that you are among people who also have problems; you no longer have that feeling of being all alone. Confidence builds up in helping and supporting each other. Finally, group therapy is relatively cheap; this makes it good value for money.

Although you do not get as much attention as in individual therapy, the advantages of group interaction more than make up for this. Treatment may last from only a few months up to several years.

7. Self-help groups and peer support. Informal therapy takes place in groups where people facing the same kind of problems meet in order to give each other support and encouragement. Some groups are organized along the pattern of Alcoholics Anonymous (one of the pioneers of self-help groups) with a "Twelve-Step" route to recovery. In this plan, participants attend regular meetings where they make a commitment to a series of twelve declarations promulgated by the group that are designed to instill a positive attitude.

From time to time everyone gets up in front of the group and reports on his (her) progress. They may sound frightening but in practice the atmosphere is designed to be so encouraging and supportive that members admire and applaud those who speak out. In turn they are encouraged to work hard at the goals they have set themselves. They look forward to reporting their own progress to the group when it comes to their own turn to address it.

About fifteen million Americans attend self-help groups every week. A popular and successful form of therapy, it provides a great feeling of community and mutual support, and a wonderful source of mutual support and shared practical advice. (If you have watched the movie "A Man Loves a Woman" which describes a wife's fight against alcoholism, then you will understand this perfectly.)

> *A friend is someone who knows all about you but likes you anyway.*
>
> Anonymous

Another great advantage is that self-help groups cost nothing or virtually nothing to participate in. Groups exist to help depression and the two major, unfortunate side effects of depression: alcoholism and substance abuse.

Some groups (or even chapters within groups) are much better run and directed than others. Attend a few meetings and check the experiences of people who have been attending for some time.

Self-help is not a substitute for severely depressed people who need medication or professional care. The best approach is to first obtain a good, professional evaluation and a recommended course of treatment (whether medication and/or therapy). Subsequently, joining a self-help group will be a good option. This is the quickest and most efficient route to recovery.

A complete list of self-help groups can be obtained from the American Self-Help Clearinghouse at Northwest Covenant Medical Center, 25 Pocono Road, Denville, New Jersey, NJ 07834 (tel. 201-625-7101). The appendix contains a state-by-state list of groups useful for depression, alcoholism, substance abuse, etc.

If the idea of a self-help group attracts you, then read also the advice in the chapter entitled "Self-help ... 205 Ways to Alleviate Depression."

If at first you don't succeed, try, try again. Then quit. No use being a damn fool about it.

W. C. Fields (1880–1946)

Chapter 12

Medications for Depression

Medicines for mental health depression were discovered by accident in the early 1950s when doctors administered the drug imipramine to treat tuberculosis in patients who happened to be depressed. To their surprise, the patients' moods improved markedly. At that time, the doctors did not understand why this happened. Nowadays, they know that it was because the drug acted beneficially on the neurotransmitters in the brain. Since then more and more drugs have been discovered to counter depression and other mental disorders.

Not every patient with depression will respond to any particular drug. Fortunately, there is now a panoply of drugs available. Therefore, if one drug does not work, a person can easily switch to another. Approximately 90% of depressed people respond to one drug or another.

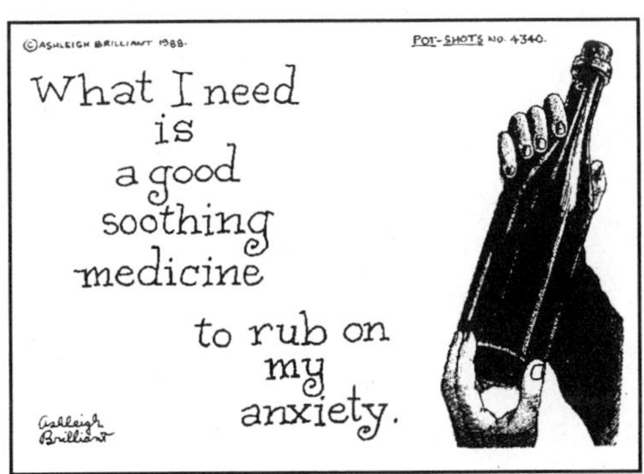

Some people experience unpleasant side effects with certain drugs. For example, nausea, dizziness, headaches, dry mouth, etc. These often diminish as the body gets used to the medication. Since there is no way of predicting how a certain medicine will affect you, you have to try it out and see. Generally speaking, the newer drugs have fewer side effects. For example, 50% of the people taking Prozac (fluoxetine) experience no side effects at all. Serzone (nefazodone), available only since 1995, is reported to have even fewer side effects. It is worth asking your doctor to have you try them out first.

A physical examination is advisable to make sure that a prescribed drug will not worsen an existing illness or condition. The doctor should also ask you which drugs you are currently taking to make sure they will not interact dangerously with the antidepressant.

Although even trained psychiatrists cannot predict with certainty which drug(s) will work best for you, there are two cases when they can make an informed guess. A drug which a family relative took for depression and which worked will probably work for you, too. The same will apply to a drug you took successfully during a previous episode of depression.

You should respond well to a drug within about eight weeks. In fact, significant, partial improvements are usually noticeable within the first two weeks. A drug is unsuitable if it produces no change whatsoever or side effects that are too unpleasant. In that case, it is time to try out a different medicine. A medicine which works for you should be found within two or three attempts in the vast majority of cases.

To dream of the person you would like to be is to waste the person you are.

Anonymous

It often happens that the right drug is prescribed in too small quantities. The result is only a partial improvement, even after eight weeks, and a switch is made to another medicine. This is a mistake, especially if there are few or no unpleasant side effects. Before giving up on such a drug, ask your psychiatrist whether the dosage can be increased.

Eight weeks may seem an unbearably long time to wait for a large improvement when you are suffering greatly. Unfortunately, there are no quicker medicines available at the present time, so keep on taking the medicine and hang in there!

Strictly speaking, medicines do not "cure" depression in the same way that antibiotics cure infectious diseases. By killing the germs, antibiotics rid the body of the illness completely. This is what doctors call a "cure." Antidepressants, on the other hand, put right the biochemistry in the brain. Once a person stops taking the medicine, the biochemical imbalance may return again. However, if the person continues to takes the medicine, perhaps in a small "maintenance" dose, the imbalance does not return. Psychiatrists say that the medicine "manages the symptoms."

The same is true for people with diabetes and high blood pressure. Their medicines only manage the symptoms; they do not rid the body of the illness. If they stop taking the medicine, the illness comes back. But while they keep to the medicine, they will not be ill and can enjoy their lives with nothing to fear.

Unfortunately, there is still a stigma about taking medicines for depression which is completely undeserved. It makes patients eager to discontinue treatment at the earliest opportunity so that they can tell the world that the illness is behind them. For the reasons explained above, this is a big mistake. The illness **can** return. In fact, people recovering from dysthymia (mild, continuous depression), severe depression, or a history of depressive attacks are at particular risk. If this applies to you, discuss with your doctor whether you can take a regular maintenance dose as an insurance against another attack. Do not let your health be put at risk by what other people may or may not think about you.

Drugs used to treat depression can be divided into three classes:

1. Tricyclic antidepressants (TCAs). Advantages: These have been found particularly effective for treating depression linked with panic attacks and (sometimes) obsessive-compulsive disorder. They are the preferred line for treatment for severe, agitated, major depressions.

   Disadvantages: Unsuitable for those with heart disease or urinary problems. There is a bad interaction with alcohol, antihypertensive medicines, sedatives, thyroid drugs, oral contraceptives, and drugs to thin blood. Smokers may require a higher dosage. An overdose can result in heart failure or fibrillations, and possible death. (Great caution is required by doctors when prescribing to suicidal patients.)

2. Monoamine oxidase inhibitors (MAOIs). Advantages: Despite the disadvantages described below, these drugs are very effective for some people, particularly those with atypical depression and depression linked to phobias and anxiety.

Disadvantages: A serious drawback is that MAOIs have a dangerous interaction with certain types of food (e.g., hard cheese, salami, corned beef, beans) which contain a substance called tyramine. The result is hypertensive crisis, a sudden rise in blood pressure which may be fatal. Symptoms include an intense, pounding headache, heart palpitations, chest pain and dizziness. An onset requires immediate emergency treatment at hospital.

For this reason, patients on MAOIs must keep off foods like cheese, salami, corned beef and beans. There is also a poor reaction to alcohol, sedatives and anti-anxiety drugs, although not to the same extent as TCAs.

A fatal reaction also can also occur when MAOIs are taken together with certain of the newer antidepressants (described below) such as Prozac, Zoloft and Wellbutrin. A large overdose is also dangerous. MAOIs may also be fatal when combined with certain pain medications (e.g., Demerol).

The effects described above last for up to two weeks after discontinuing an MAOI and patients should be just as careful during this period.

3. Newer antidepressants, including selective serotonin reuptake inhibitors (SSRIs). Advantages: Discovered in the late 1980s, these drugs have generally fewer and safer side effects than TCAs and MAOIs. For example, half of those who take Prozac (fluoxetine) do not experience any side effects. An overdose is not dangerous. They generally produce weight loss rather than weight gain, an important consideration to those watching their figures.

The hypertensive and heart risk is negligible and there is no need for a special diet. Some of these drugs may also be helpful in treating obsessive-compulsive disorder and bulimia.

Disadvantages: Side effects such as irritability and agitation occur in a minority of patients but often diminish with time. Other medicines can be taken to combat these side effects.

Overall, these are the safest and most effective antidepressants.

COMMONLY PRESCRIBED ANTIDEPRESSANTS		
Tricyclics (TCAs)	**Monoamine Oxidase Inhibitors (MAOIs)**	**Newer Anti-depressants (Excluding SSRIs)**
Amitriptyline (Elavil, Endep)	Isocarboxazid (Marplan)	Amoxapine (Asendin)
Clomipramine (Anafranil)	Phenelzine (Nardil)	Bupropion (Wellbutrin)
Desipramine (Norpramin)	Tranylcypromine (Parnate)	Maprotiline (Ludiomil)
Doxepin (Adapin, Sinequan)	**Selective Serotonin Reuptake Inhibitors (SSRIs)**	Nefazodone (Serzone)
Imipramine (Tofranil)	Fluoxetine (Prozac)	Trazodone (Desyrel)
Nortriptyline (Pamelor)	Fluvoxamine (Luvox)	Venlafaxine (Effexor)
Protriptyline (Vivactil)	Paroxetine (Paxil)	
Trimipramine (Surmontil)	Sertraline (Zoloft)	
N.B. Trade names are in parentheses.		

There is another set of drugs used mainly to treat people with manic depression (bipolar depression). They reduce or protect against recurring attacks of mania and depression. Although they are also effective against depression alone (unipolar depression), they are rarely made the first choice for this purpose. Therefore, they have been put here into a fourth class:

4. Drugs for bipolar (manic-depressive) disorder. Advantages: Good for treating acute, severe episodes of depression (particularly in patients whose moods change rapidly). These drugs are often used successfully in conjunction with other anti-depressants to which a patient does not respond when used alone.

Disadvantages: Lithium (the most well known) and the other drugs may produce annoying side effects, including memory problems. A large overdose can be dangerous. Long term use may damage a person's thyroid function. Blood levels have to be routinely measured to check the concentration of the drug and prevent adverse effects. This may be a nuisance. People taking lithium also need to drink plenty of water and keep their salt intake steady.

OTHER DRUGS USED AGAINST DEPRESSION

Used Mainly for Manic Depression

Lithium (Various brands)	Carbamazepine (Tegretol)	Valproate (Depakote, Depakene)

N.B. Trade names in parentheses.

For further helpful and detailed information about drugs for depression, see References and Sources (page 163).

WHY AN ANTI-DEPRESSANT MAY FAIL

1. Too small a dose
2. Not taken long enough
3. Not the right drug; try another
4. Depression responds better to psychotherapy than to drugs
5. Depression does not respond to any treatment (very rare)

Now is the time that people will refer to years from now when they say, "In the good old days ..."

Anonymous

Chapter 13

Other Treatments

Psychotherapy and medications are the most usual treatments for depression. However, other mainstream approaches exist: electroconvulsive therapy, phototherapy, and biofeedback.

1. Electroconvulsive therapy (ECT). When a patient is severely depressed and potentially suicidal, this form of treatment is a viable option. The same is true when a depressed patient has tried all sorts of other treatments and none have worked. Other treatments are usually preferred for patients who are only mildly depressed.

POT-SHOTS NO. 4614
BEAUTY IS ONLY SKIN DEEP
BUT FORTUNATELY, I HAVE VERY DEEP SKIN.
Ashleigh Brilliant
© ASHLEIGH BRILLIANT 1988.

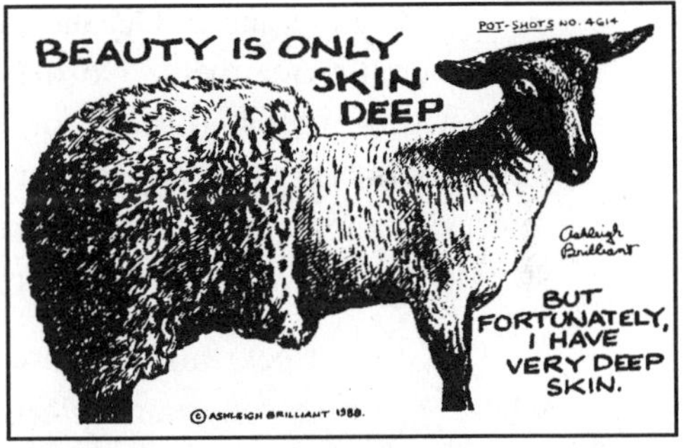

The patient is sedated with a general anesthetic and a muscle relaxant. An electric current is passed in carefully controlled pulses between two electrodes (electrical contacts) which are attached to the patient's head. The electric pulses induce brief seizures in the brain which cause the depression to lift. Apparently the biochemical imbalances are corrected, although scientific researchers do not as yet understand exactly how this works.

During this operation, which lasts from 20 to 40 minutes, the patient feels absolutely nothing. There are no sudden or violent jerks of the body or limbs when the current pulses are applied. Sometimes the fingers and toes move slightly but that is about all. Treatments are administered two or three times a week up to a total of six to twelve treatments in all.

When the electroconvulsive therapy was first developed, the technique was unrefined and often badly applied. Sometimes serious complications developed such as violent body movements, bone fractures, heart seizures, etc. Movies and books sensationalized the stories and gave the treatment a bad name. Nowadays, however, the treatment has been much improved and is very safe and effective owing to careful monitoring. Therefore, there is no need for concern like there used to be.

Advantages: Recovery is relatively rapid, taking only a few weeks. This is advantageous for the severely depressed, especially those in danger of suicide. There is no trial and error process as with medications and psychotherapy. Painful mental anguish associated with depression rapidly diminishes. The patient can go on to rebuild his (her) life sooner than with other treatments.

Disadvantages: Occasionally there is temporary memory loss after the treatment. Normally, memory returns to normal after a few weeks. (On the other hand, a severely depressed patient who opts for longer term treatment will also experience poorer memory due to poor concentration, as explained in the section about symptoms of depression.)

Side effects may include headaches, slight skin burns where the electrodes are placed, mild muscle soreness, or nausea. These disappear after a number of weeks.

2. Phototherapy (light therapy). Approximately, 10 million people (4% of the population in the USA) suffer from seasonal affective disorder (SAD). They experience periods of sadness during the winter but not during the summer. Researchers believe the cause is connected to the shortness of daylight in winter. Exposing such people to bright, artificial light has been found to lift the depression. Apparently, the biological clock is fooled into thinking that the hours of daylight are longer than they actually are.

The patient sits in front of a bank of very bright lights for about thirty minutes during the evening or very early in the morning when it is still dark. After two or three days the depression starts to lift.

Latest research has found an even easier solution: a computerized dawn simulator called "Sphere Daylight." As the patient sleeps, this gadget emits low-intensity light a few hours before dawn which penetrates closed eyelids and persuades the brain that winter has passed and spring has arrived. This machine has been invented by the New York State Psychiatric Institute at Columbia University (Winter Depression Program). It can be obtained from SphereOne, 20 Easedale Road, Wayne, NJ 07470 (tel. 201-942-9772) at a cost of approximately $360.

Advantages: Rapid recovery and no known side effects, provided that the eyes are properly protected during treatment.

Disadvantages: None. Unfortunately, this treatment works only for the minority whose depression comes under the category of seasonal affective disorder.

3. Biofeedback. A process where a person can gain conscious control over his (her) emotional and physiological states. For example, an anxious person can learn to relax. A person who finds it hard to fall asleep at night can learn to do so. This kind of treatment is suitable only for someone who is mildly depressed.

The patient is connected to sensitive electrical equipment which monitors pulse, blood pressure, perspiration, skin temperature, muscle tension and brain waves. The therapist encourages him (her) to imagine that the pulse is decreased, muscles are relaxed, thoughts are more placid, and so on. Thinking thus can change the physical state of the body.

As the electrical equipment detects changes in the tension of the muscles, temperature of the skin, rate of heart beat, brain waves, etc., it emits a series of beeps or light flashes. The patient knows that the thoughts processes are working and remembers them for the future. (Hence the name "feedback.") By this method, learning becomes more and more automatic. Eventually, the patient can calm himself (herself) whenever he (she) feels anxious. At night he (she) can "think" himself (herself) to sleep.

Only biofeedback therapists accredited by the Biofeedback Certification Institute of America (BCIA), 10200 West 44 Avenue, Suite 304, Wheat Ridge, CO 80033 (tel. 303-420-2902) should be consulted.

Advantages: Treatment is fairly rapid, taking only about a week to learn the process of relaxation. Good for someone who has experienced a temporary upset, e.g. a family bereavement, producing anxiety and other physical symptoms.

Disadvantages: Effect may be only temporary or may not work in very stressful situations. Not recommended for those with severe depression, recurring depression or mild, continuous depression (dysthymia) for whom medications and/or psychotherapy are preferable.

> *Victory belongs to the most persevering.*
>
> Napoleon Bonaparte (1769–1821)

Chapter 14

Nutritional Healing and Drug-free Remedies

This chapter discusses nutritional healing, herbal remedies, aromatherapy, logotherapy, music therapy, and color therapy.

A view growing in popularity among the general public is that modern life with junk foods, alcohol and drug abuse, pollution, fast-paced stress, etc. is throwing our health out of balance. To make matters worse, we rely too much on artificially manufactured drugs to cure our physical and mental ills. Instead, we should allow nature to utilize the healing forces from within our own bodies in conjunction with the right naturally occurring substances.

A popular and useful book written on this subject is "Prescription for Nutritional Healing" by James F. Balch, M.D., and Phyllis A. Balch, C.N.C., who have had widespread experience in nutritional healing. According to these experts, this type of healing should be used in conjunction with mainstream medical treatment, and always under the supervision of a trained professional. This applies particularly to depression, a serious condition which can rapidly worsen and go out of control with the wrong or ineffective treatment.

Therefore, if you are interested in nutritional healing, let your doctor know. If he (she) prescribes a manufactured drug to combat depression, do not reject it. This does not mean you have to give up on nutritional healing, On the contrary, use it at the same time to speed up your recovery and lessen any side effects.

Certain ingredients of naturally occurring foods are good for combatting depression owing to their beneficial effect on the brain's neurotransmitters. Complex carbohydrates have a calming effect while proteins increase alertness. However, foods high in saturated fats should be avoided as they lead to fatigue, slow thinking and sluggishness.

(Simple carbohydrates result in a quick rush of energy followed by fatigue and depression and, therefore, are not recommended.)

Tyrosine is good for reducing prolonged, intense or uncontrollable stress. However, it should **not** be taken if you are on monoamine oxidase inhibitor (MAOI) drugs as the combination can raise the blood pressure to dangerous levels and cause nasty headaches.

If you choose to follow a nutritional diet to help conquer your depression, include the following ingredients:

1. proteins; e.g., turkey, salmon, and white fish
2. complex carbohydrates; e.g., whole wheat bread, raw fruit, vegetables, and soybeans

Exclude the following substances:

1. highly saturated fats; e.g., fried foods, pork, hamburgers
2. phenylalanine if you experience anxiety attacks
3. choline, ornithine, and arginine if you have manic depression (bipolar disorder)
4. tyrosine if you are taking MAOIs; e.g., cheese, chocolate, herring, yogurt, wine, beer, and yeast
5. caffeine (except in small quantities)

Recommended nutrients (unless excluded above) are:

1. vitamin B complex (100 mg. three times daily)
2. choline and inositol or lecithin (100 mg. twice daily)
3. gerovital H-3 (for people over 35 years old)
4. L-tyrosine (approximately 100 mg. per kg. of body weight; take daily with 1,000 mg. of vitamin C and 50 mg. of vitamin B_6 at least three hours after eating any food)
5. niacin (B_3) (100 mg. three times daily)
6. melatonin (2 mg. at bedtime) for seasonal affective disorder (SAD)
7. D-phenylalanine (500 or 1,000 mg. three times daily)

Other helpful supplements are: aslavitol (particularly beneficial for the elderly), calcium, magnesium, gamma-amino butyric acid, lithium arginate or orotate (for manic depression), multivitamin and mineral complex, zinc chelate, chromium, primrose or black currant oil, spirulina and crude bee pollen. Take these (or some of these) after discussion with your mental health practitioner, and avoid if included in the exclusions above.

Eat a breakfast that includes a serving of grain, fresh food, and low-fat dairy food. Consume several small meals and snacks distributed throughout the day instead of having your food in three large meals. This will maintain a constant high level of energy and make you less prone to fatigue, insomnia, and depression. Drink plenty of water; low-grade dehydration is a common cause of fatigue. Finally, talk to your doctor about your diet before changing it.

Herbs are also useful natural remedies. Top on the list are ginkgo and St. John's wort, obtainable in the form of tablets, capsules, and extracts. Numerous clinical trials show that ginkgo helps alleviate short-term memory loss and depression. However, it should not be taken in excess because overlarge doses may cause restlessness, stomach upset, diarrhea, and vomiting. A European study reveals that St. John's wort is just as effective (for mild depression) as the anti-depressants imipramine and maprotiline, and has fewer side effects. However, it is a stimulant and makes the skin sensitive to sunlight. Therefore, this herb should not be taken at night and sunbathing should be avoided.

Chamomile (teas, ointments, lotions, and inhalations) is a mild sedative. Ginseng (teas, powders, capsules, tablets, and extracts) is said to build up the body's resistance to stress. Valerian is a minor tranquilizer for reducing restlessness and sleep disturbances. Except in rare cases, all three have insignificant side effects.

Aromatherapy, treatment by fragrant oils, containing highly concentrated substances produced by aromatic plants or trees, has recently grown in popularity. Lavender brings on calmness and induces sleep. Peppermint increases alertness. A mixture of ylang-ylang, marjoram, and jasmine oils are claimed to heighten self-confidence.

Inhalation is not the only method of treatment; these oils can also be used in steam preparations, applied in compresses, soaked up in the bathtub, or diffused through a room. No controlled scientific studies of aromatherapy and its effectiveness in treating depression have yet been conducted.

Logotherapy is treatment by reading self-help and improvement books. A recent study shows it may be helpful to people with mild to moderate depression (dysthymia). The elderly and others who have lots of time on their hands (and even those who do not) could try out this approach. Presumably the same result can be obtained from watching motivational videos and movies, and listening to inspirational audio cassette tapes. Those who have little time or patience to read will naturally prefer this approach!

Many people find listening to music very soothing. Music therapy can help lift sad moods and improve general mental health. Research indicates that, like exercise, it causes the brain to release endorphins, pain-killing hormones which help brighten a person's mood. Soft music, in particular, alleviates stress and promotes relaxation. On the other hand, loud, discordant music and mournful tunes should be avoided.

Color is known to have an effect on people's moods. According to Dr. Alexander Schauss, director of the American Institute for Biosocial Research in Tacoma, Washington, light energy stimulates the pituitary and pineal glands. These affect the production of hormones and the functioning of other physiological systems. Therefore, colors around you (e.g., in the home and office) affect the way you feel and think.

Color therapy means choosing a combination of colors in your surroundings that make you feel happiest, brightest, and most productive. Keep this in mind when buying wallpaper, paint, furniture, and clothes. Red stimulates, pink tranquilizes and soothes anxiety, orange stimulates the appetite and reduces fatigue, and blue has a calming effect. The best colors for easing depression overall appear to be green and yellow. Green soothes and relaxes; yellow energizes, lifts the spirits, and boosts memory power.

Advantages of drug-free remedies: A useful supplement to mainstream drugs, and a healthy way of living. May speed up recovery and reduce side effects.

Disadvantages: None. These remedies should not be considered a replacement for mainstream drugs.

> *Happiness is good health and a bad memory.*
>
> Ingrid Bergman (1915–1982)

Chapter 15

How to Choose a Treatment Practitioner

It is very important to find someone whom you can be confident will make a correct diagnosis and recommend the right treatment first time. You want to feel happy and comfortable with life as soon as possible, and do not want to waste your time and money on someone who makes a mistake or is not competent. But how does one find such a person?

©ASHLEIGH BRILLIANT 1983.
POT-SHOTS NO. 3154.
Somehow, I have to play my role in life as a gifted, beautiful, happy, well-adjusted person.
Ashleigh Brilliant

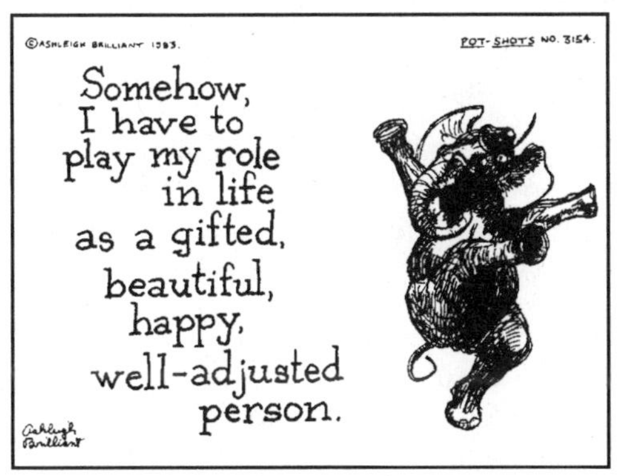

Pick up any newspaper or magazine and you will find advertisements for psychiatrists and therapists promising cures for all mental ills ranging from depression through anxieties and phobias to smoking, eating and drinking addictions. You envisage a long course of therapy, possibly in combination with psychiatric drugs. Other advertisements may recommend homeopathic remedies, using naturally occurring substances. (The "National Examiner" had an article [December 12, 1995] recommending a "miracle cocktail" of garlic, apple cider vinegar, and honey!) At the same time, your family physician may recommend vitamins, tranquilizers, exercise and a vacation. You sift through all these and feel very confused. Which treatment is right for you and what should you do?

The best thing to do is consult with an expert who is highly experienced and familiar with depression and other forms of mental illness. He should be knowledgeable about the various treatments available, and able to tailor a treatment for each individual. For an initial diagnosis you cannot go wrong by seeing a psychiatrist who is a medical doctor with specialized training in mental disorders, and the only specialist authorized to prescribe psychiatric drugs.

Find someone who has a solid reputation. Listen to advice from friends and relatives, and seek referrals from your family physician. Above all, choose someone who has a record of many successes; do not rely on only one or two success stories. (The author wishes it were easy to take up references from former patients. After all, this is common practice in other professions, e.g., accountants, lawyers, and builders where one invests a lot of time and money. Unfortunately, the rules of confidentiality between doctor and patient may get in the way, making it impossible, therefore, to obtain these important references.)

Suppose that your friends, relatives and family physician are unable to refer you to a good specialist, or that you do not want to take any chances. In that case there is a list of psychiatrists who are widely recognized as being eminent in their field.

You can ask your family physician to make an initial contact with one of these psychiatrists who is close to your local area. (This is the best way since these specialists are extremely busy and may have questions about your case that only your doctor can answer.)

Although the psychiatrist will most likely be too busy to see you, he (she) will be able to refer you to another specialist whom he (she) knows personally and is, therefore, bound to be competent. Alternatively, the psychiatrist's secretary can make the referral. The list is printed in the References and Sources (page 171).

It is not recommended that you scan through the "Yellow Pages" in your telephone directory and pick a psychiatrist (or other mental health practitioner) at random because the directory does not screen those it lists.

A later chapter (see page 103) deals with obtaining free or cheap treatment.

> *To be successful, you have to keep moving. After all, no one stumbles on something sitting down.*
>
> Anonymous

Chapter 16

The First Visit

What should you expect to happen? Is the psychiatrist right for you? This section deals with these questions.

Although you must trust the psychiatrist for technical expertise, you should make a judgement based on his (her) general manner. Overall you should feel that he (she) is competent, friendly, warm and concerned; a person who is able to put you at ease and encourage you to ask questions. It is a bad sign if he (she) is authoritarian and condescending, however well recommended. If so, it is best to look for someone else.

This is what you should expect to happen during the first visit. When referred to the psychiatrist, it is natural to wonder and perhaps worry about what will happen during the evaluation. You may feel uncomfortable about revealing personal details about yourself to a stranger (even though that stranger is a doctor). Or you may feel ashamed to admit difficulty in handling your problems on your own. You may worry that the therapist will judge you negatively or conclude that your symptoms mean that you are "crazy."

POT-SHOTS NO 2770.
BY WHAT PROCESS DID I BECOME A STRANGER IN MY OWN LIFE?

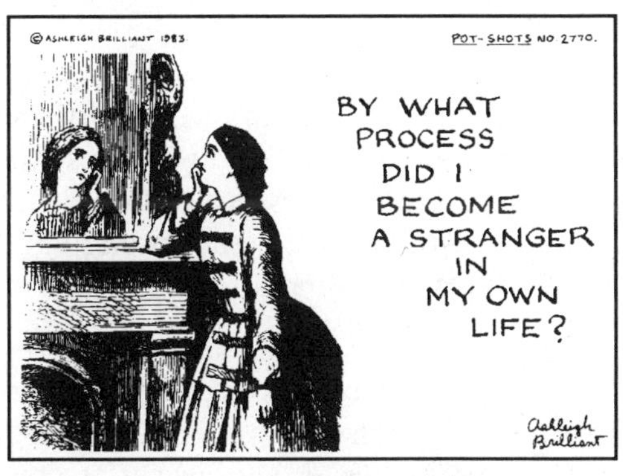

Do not worry; these feelings are all perfectly normal. Psychiatrists know this and will not look down on you. In fact, they will have seen lots of people like yourself before and probably some with even worse problems. Their job is to help, to listen, and to direct a suitable course of treatment. In order to assist them and get the most out of treatment, follow these guidelines:

1. Be honest, truthful and open, so that the specialist can assess the problem correctly. Do not keep secrets.

2. Express your thoughts and feelings freely.

3. Be confident in the specialist's professional abilities, realizing that he (she) has treated many patients with similar problems and is an expert in human behavior.

4. Do not be concerned with the impression you are making. You will not lose respect or concern in the eyes of the specialist, no matter how difficult or troubling your problem is.

5. As you reveal your problems, you may feel powerful emotions, such as intense anger, bitterness or sadness. Do not be embarrassed to talk about these emotions. It is good for the specialist to know how you are feeling, and doing so is often a therapy in itself.

Nothing will ever be attempted without overcoming the initial hesitation.

Anonymous

6. Prepare a written or mental list of questions to ask the specialist. Add the following to this list: "What is your opinion about my problem? Is it an illness? If so, what kind of treatment are you thinking of recommending? What are the risks, complications, benefits, and costs?"

7. Don't feel ashamed or embarrassed if you find it difficult to talk. Discussing emotionally charged details commonly arouses intense anxiety. Even the most articulate person may find it impossible to talk clearly or concisely. Take your time.

8. Do not be afraid that your problems will be revealed to someone else. The specialist will respect your confidentiality and will reveal details only with your prior written consent. This is his (her) legal, moral and professional duty. The only exception is if your life appears to be in immediate danger; for example, you may shortly commit suicide.

The specialist will observe your emotional functioning, your cognitive ability (thinking and reasoning), and your general physical state. Aspects of these will include:

1. Appearance. This can provide diagnostic hints to your state of mind. For example, people who are depressed usually pay little attention to their dress and grooming. (This does not mean that **all** untidy people are depressed.) Also, some physical illnesses which affect the mood (e.g., Graves' disease, a thyroid disorder) have distinctive physical characteristics.

2. Behavior. Typical behaviors often mark specific disorders. For example, depression is characterized by lethargy and self-deprecation. Mania (the "up" phase of bipolar disorder) is indicated by fast and high-spirited activity.

3. Speaking manner. Rapid and pressured speech indicates mania and/or bipolar disorder, while a flat, lifeless monotone indicates depression.

4. Affect. This term refers to the type, intensity and duration of emotion a person displays externally. Depressed people exhibit continual sadness, guilt and hopelessness. Anxiousness and apprehensiveness are also common. Mania is marked by euphoria and bipolar disorder by rapidly shifting spirits.

   The specialist will assess the intensity and duration of the emotions displayed and whether they are consistent with that expected in a normal situation.

5. Thought processes. The way you structure thoughts and reach conclusions is important to the evaluation process. Do you think logically and can you describe events and their relationship to problems clearly? How good is your concentration?

6. Thought content. Are your thoughts marked by delusions (beliefs that are objectively incorrect and out of keeping with your background) and/or obsessions (ideas which you recognize as irrational that keep intruding into your mind)?

   For example, depression is often marked by obsessive attention to detail and perfection. Psychotically depressed people may be convinced that they are equivalent to garbage in worth.

7. Intellectual function. Depression slows down the ability to calculate, think abstractly, and use words correctly. It often masks underlying intelligence.

8. Memory. The specialist will assess both your short-term and long-term memory. Depression often impairs memory, especially short-term memory. (A physical illness that influences brain functioning may also affect memory.)

9. Orientation. A psychotically depressed person may be so disoriented as to be unaware of such facts as the date, the time, or the name of the president.

10. Insight. This term refers to the extent of a person's self-understanding. Some people with depression understand that they are suffering from an emotional disorder. Others acknowledge that they are ill but blame this on other people or uncontrollable events.

    On the other hand, people in the manic phase of bipolar disorder are typically convinced that they are not ill and completely deny that a problem exists.

11. General physical state. The specialist's evaluation will include a medical history and a physical examination to see if an underlying physical illness is causing or contributing to the depression or mood disorder. The physical examination may be carried out by another specialist.

    Depression is usually accompanied by physical complaints. For example, appetite and sleep changes and gastrointestinal disturbances are common. Conversely, many physical conditions (ranging from thyroid disorders to brain tumors and including such illnesses as Parkinson's disease and Huntington's chorea) can cause psychiatric symptoms such as depression.

12. Family history. The specialist will ask whether other members of your family have had depression and/or bipolar disorder. This may provide an important clue since these illnesses have a hereditary disposition.

> *Where the willingness is great, the difficulties cannot be great.*
>
> Niccolo Machiavelli (1469–1527)

Chapter 17

Subsequent Visits

As the treatment progresses, how can you remain confident in your choice of mental health practitioner? Treatment is very much an individualized process. Generally speaking, you should feel comfortable (allowing for a few brief ups and downs) with the practitioner, free to ask questions and discuss doubts, and find that you are gradually making improvements. Every month or so, ask yourself the following questions:

1. Do you feel comfortable talking about your problems?
2. Are your questions answered or ignored or sidestepped?
3. Do you feel you are being treated seriously?
4. Is the practitioner someone whom you respect and trust?
5. Have clear treatment goals been set and are they being followed?
6. Do you understand the roles of both yourself and the practitioner?
7. Has the usual course of treatment been explained clearly to you and is it basically being followed?
8. Have the side effects of any medication(s) you are taking and how to cope with them been explained to you?
9. Do you notice any improvements?
10. Is the practitioner keen on achieving recovery targets within the time goals set?
11. Are there regular progress reviews?

12. If there is no improvement, have you been taking the medication(s) as prescribed and/or doing the recommended therapeutic exercises? How does the practitioner explain this? What does he (she) suggest?

13. If you are recovering, is a schedule for reducing and/or discontinuing treatment being worked out?

Although you may not have exact and definite answers to all of these questions, you should be generally satisfied with the information you do have. Otherwise, you should consider asking for another course of treatment and/or changing practitioner.

I walk slowly but I never walk backwards.

Abraham Lincoln (1809–1865)

Chapter 18

How Effective is the Treatment? Is it Working?

What does "effective" treatment mean? First of all, how do you measure the amount or proportion of recovery? Then in what time scale and at what cost? The problem is that any improvement is very subjective.

On the one hand, with a physical illness like influenza, you know you are well when your temperature is down to normal, the coughing has stopped, your headache has gone, and your throat no longer hurts. In the case of hypertension (too high blood pressure), you know when you are well when your blood pressure has dropped down to normal. On the other hand, with an emotional illness like depression, how do you measure "feeling happier"? And how much happier do you have to be in order to be well? If only there could be invented a happiness "thermometer"!

In the absence of such an instrument, you have to use subjective measurements and rules of thumb. Below is an example of a chart to track recovery at regular intervals (e.g., daily or weekly), which your psychiatrist or therapist should construct with you and tailor to your personal circumstances.

Using this chart to measure your progress, you can assess whether your treatment is working, whether you should try a different line of medication, or whether you should change your psychotherapist. Allow up to six to ten weeks to assess the effectiveness of medication, and three to six months to assess whether a course of psychotherapy is working.

(Some psychotherapists will argue that it can take up to a year before recovery becomes apparent. The author believes that this is not good enough. Considering the time and money you are investing, you need results faster than this. Moreover, even if recovery does take a full year (and there is never any guarantee), you should be able to see some results within a few months.)

Many mental health practitioners do not use such charts and may feel uncomfortable with them. You should explain to your practitioner that charting and assessing your progress is important to you. If he (she) is still unwilling to use a progress chart, it is a bad sign. It could indicates that he (she) has had poor success in the past and is afraid of being found out. Or he (she) may be planning to have you (and your fees) on the books for a long time. Taking a risk like this is unwise and it would be better to switch to another practitioner who is willing to be accountable and for whom speed of recovery is important.

CHART TO TRACK RECOVERY: AN EXAMPLE

Month: June 199x	**1**	**2**	**3**	**4**	**5**
Physical symptoms: Sleep					
How many hours do you sleep?					
How many times do you wake up during the night?					
How long does it take for you to fall asleep?					
How early in the morning do you wake up?					
Do you feel so tired during the day that you doze off? If so, how often and for how long?					
Physical symptoms: Appetite					
Do you overeat? How often?					
Do you undereat? How often?					
Have you been gaining or losing weight?					
How often do you eat a snack (e.g., candies) because you feel miserable?					
Any diarrhea or constipation?					

CHART TO TRACK RECOVERY: AN EXAMPLE

Month: June 199x	1	2	3	4	5
Physical symptoms: Fatigue					
Do you feel so exhausted that you have to drag yourself through the day? How many hours?					
Does this disrupt your work?					
Do you wake up unrefreshed?					
Physical symptoms: Anhedonia					
Do you experience any pleasure? For how long? (This is a comparative guide.)					
Do you feel a zest for life? (Put on a scale of 1 through 10.)					
Are you doing any activities you used to lose interest in?					
Physical symptoms: Panic attacks					
Do you experience any panic attacks, feeling of losing control, etc.? How often?					
Physical symptoms: Miscellaneous					
Any headaches? For how long?					
Sickness or nausea? For how long?					
Any symptoms without any physical basis?					
Emotional symptoms: Sadness					
How miserable do you feel? (Enter on a scale of 1 through 10.)					
Do you break down into tears? How often?					
Do you feel a pit at the bottom of your stomach? For how long?					
Emotional symptoms: Self-esteem. (Enter the following on a scale of 1 through 10.) Do you:					
feel worthless?					

CHART TO TRACK RECOVERY: AN EXAMPLE					
Month: June 199x	**1**	**2**	**3**	**4**	**5**
hate yourself?					
feel you have to please everybody?					
feel inferior to others?					
find it difficult to persuade others of your views?					
usually defer to the opinions of other people even when you disagree?					
Emotional symptoms: Apathy. (Enter the following on a scale of 1 through 10.)					
Do you feel little interest in life?					
How easy is it to arouse enthusiasm in something?					
Do you have a good social life? Do you sometimes stay indoors rather than mix with others?					
Emotional symptoms: Interpersonal problems. (Enter the following on a scale of 1 through 10.)					
When criticized or rejected: (a) how hurt do you feel?					
(b) how long (days or hours) does it take for you to bounce back?					
How comfortable do you feel around other people?					
Do you frequently feel very lonely?					
Are you often unreasonably irritable?					
Emotional symptoms: Guilt feelings. (Enter the following on a scale of 1 through 10.)					
Do you feel excessively or continually guilty or remorseful?					
Do you feel excessively or continually bad about yourself?					

CHART TO TRACK RECOVERY: AN EXAMPLE

Month: June 199x	1	2	3	4	5
Emotional symptoms: Negative thinking. (Enter the following on a scale of 1 through 10.)					
Is it hard to feel positive or optimistic about things in general?					
Emotional symptoms: Suicidal thoughts. (Enter the following on a scale of 1 through 10.)					
How often do you feel life is not worth living?					
Do you sometimes feel like ending your life?					
Other symptoms: Concentration and memory. (Enter the following on a scale of 1 through 10.)					
How easily do you concentrate?					
How easily do you grasp what is going on around you?					
How good is your short-term memory?					
Do you forget things easily?					
Other symptoms: Hypochondria. (Enter the following on a scale of 1 through 10.)					
Are you afraid you have a dangerous illness (e.g., cancer or heart trouble)?					
Do you constantly worry about your health?					

Besides the doctor, you also have a responsibility to make sure that treatment is effective. Persevere, give the treatment a chance to work, and discuss your feelings candidly with the doctor. Make some allowance for initial fears, unrealistic expectations, and changing attitudes towards the mental health practitioner. These feelings are all natural; the main outcome is that you feel an overall satisfaction with the treatment and can see that it is working within a reasonable period of time.

Recovery can be sometimes be a painful process. This is very natural. Imagine that, because of your depression, you have been unable to face an unpleasant manager, fellow worker or school mate who has constantly been putting you down. He (she) has been a constant source of distress. Now, after taking medication for eight weeks, your spirits have lifted and you feel like trying to assert yourself. Now comes the big test. You go to work or school. The unpleasant person sees you and makes a nasty remark in front of others. You decide to answer back. Butterflies are fluttering in your stomach. A lump forms in your throat. Somehow you manage to stammer out what you have to say. The unpleasant person glares at you and you feel very awkward.

©ASHLEIGH BRILLIANT 1982.
POT-SHOTS NO. 2433.
SOMETIMES
I WISH
I COULD GIVE
ALL MY
EMOTIONS
THE DAY
OFF.
Ashleigh Brilliant

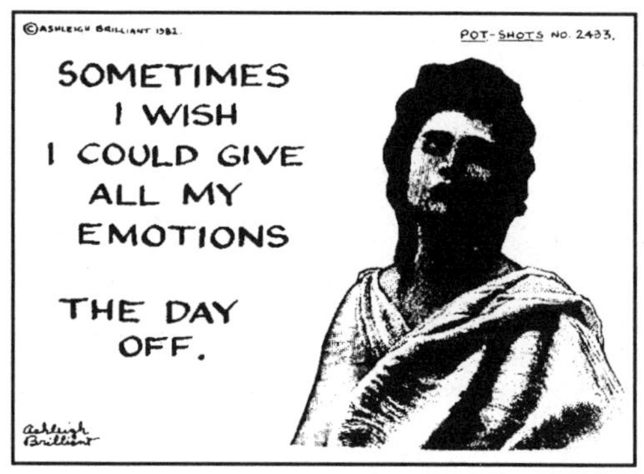

On reflection, it would have been easier to have given up and said nothing as you usually do. But, difficult and painful though it was, you managed to stand up for yourself. Next time the unpleasant person will think twice before putting you down. If he (she) makes another nasty remark, you will find it easier to stand up for yourself than last time. And next time after that even easier. Soon he (she) will not even **think** of insulting you. He (she) will hold you with more respect and so will everyone else.

Who says recovery is not a painful process? In many ways it is like recovering from a broken leg. Imagine your leg has been in plaster for six months. After examining the x-rays, the doctors declare that your bone is healed. The nurse breaks the plaster and you are now ready for physiotherapy. You try and walk a few steps and you fall over! Of course, says the physiotherapist, you have not used your leg muscles for a long time and they are very weak. You have to perform exercises in order to strengthen those muscles and teach your leg how to walk again.

The exercises begin at an easy and simple level. Gradually they get harder and harder. Sometimes, however careful you and the physiotherapist are, you overstrain the muscles. Then they hurt! Occasionally, you may fall over and have a setback from which you recover. After a few months you find you can walk and run just as you used to before the accident.

Recovery from severe or prolonged depression is similar. After taking medication for a few months, the neurotransmitter functional levels are much nearer normal. In principle, you can face the emotional slings and arrows of life. However, the "muscles" of your mind (the assertive part, that is) are weak and you have not used them for a long time. Perhaps never at all! You have to perform exercises in order to strengthen those "muscles" and teach your mind how to assert itself again.

Ideally, they begin at a simple level and gradually get harder and harder. Unlike physiotherapy, emotional "exercises" cannot be controlled. They are whatever life presents you with, and life is never predictable. Sometimes, therefore, you "trip over" and have a setback. It can be painful at times! However, as you carry on, the "exercises" get easier and easier and less and less painful.

When you eventually find that you can assert yourself strongly, win respect from yourself and from others, be successful socially, and manage to do all this without even consciously thinking about it, then you will know that the effort will have been worthwhile. It is the end result which counts.

Success is one percent inspiration and ninety-nine percent perspiration.

Thomas Edison (1847–1931)

Incidentally, concentration can be regarded as a "bellwether" of depression. The less the depression, the better and faster the concentration. An unusual but effective (and certainly most enjoyable) way of measuring your concentration objectively is by means of electronic games. For example, shooting down the invading Martians and their missiles. A scoreboard of hits is kept which can be used to measure progress from week to week. Different speeds and skill levels provide a sensitive measure of concentration. This can be one of the most objective ways of measuring recovery. A list of recommended games, playable on IBM personal computers is given in the table below:

COMPUTER GAMES TO MONITOR CONCENTRATION
Tetris. A challenge to manipulate various shapes falling from the top of the playing area and arrange them in solid rows at the bottom. When a solid row is formed, it vanishes resulting in points and the opportunity to build further rows. Various levels and speeds. Very simple to learn. A sensitive monitor of concentration. Highly recommended.
Jezz Ball. A game to build walls to trap moving, newly-discovered galactic atoms in small chambers in order to bring back to Earth. Various levels of skill and difficulty. Simple to learn. Recommended.
Rodent's Revenge. A cat-and-mouse game with a twist. You are the mouse and are trying to outsmart the cats by trapping them inside small spaces. The longer you survive, the better your concentration. Various levels of speed and difficulty. Simple to learn. Recommended.
Pipe Dream. A miracle sewage cleaner has been invented but is being produced much faster than it can be stored into containers. The challenge is to construct a system of pipes in time to carry it away to safety. A game of speed and strategy. Various levels of difficulty. Fairly simple to learn.
Chip's Challenge. The goal is to cross a room filled with various traps and counter-traps. Various levels of difficulty. Lots of items to memorize. Rather complicated to learn.
Tetra Vex. The object is to fill a grid of squares with tiles and make adjacent patterns match. Various levels of complexity.
Tri Peaks. A card game for one player. The object is to uncover and clear cards arranged in three piles. Tests memory and perseverance. Only one level of difficulty. No time targets. Takes time to learn.
N.B. The above games are all obtainable from MicroSoft as part of their "Best of Entertainment" pack. Requires Microsoft Windows 95 or 3.1 operating system.
Memory Tutor. A series of upturned cards are arranged in rows. They contain pairs of matching cards. The object is to guess and uncover the pairs with the fewest attempts. Various levels of difficulty. (For children.)
N.B. The above game is available from Titanium Seal Shareware. Requires DOS operating system.

Improvements may go on for far longer than you suspect, especially when your depression has been going on for months or years. This applies even if the depression has been only mild. Eventually you may reach a level of capability, productivity, self-respect, respect from others, etc. that you never thought or even dreamed you could ever achieve.

In other words, when you think you are "recovered," there are times when you can get even better. At this time you may only need to take maintenance medication which is relatively cheap. (Maintenance medication is particularly useful for preventing relapses in people with a history of recurrent major depression.) Improvements may come of their own accord without the need for expensive psychotherapy. It is worth persevering with the treatment for up to, say, a year until the improvements level off. Then you can be confident that you have reached your ultimate level of recovery.

> *Success can be measured more by obstacles overcome when trying to reach success than by plateaux achieved.*
>
> Anonymous

WHEN THERAPY WORKS

According to a study conducted by the University of Pennsylvania, patients who benefit most from therapy rate the following factors as most important to success (1 = unimportant; 4 = very important):

Factor		Rating
1.	Getting an understanding of the reasons behind my behavior and feelings	4.0
2.	A positive relationship with my therapist	3.8
3.	Talking about feelings that are difficult to discuss	3.8
4.	Getting a feeling of hope	3.8
5.	Becoming aware of and in touch with my feelings	3.8
6.	Getting guidance	3.6
7.	Relief from getting things off my chest	3.6
8.	Talking about my feelings towards my therapist	3.2
9.	Earning my therapist's approval	2.8
10.	Having my feelings stirred up	2.4
11.	My therapist making clear what he (she) thinks I should do in order to improve	2.2

Extracted from "Why My Therapy Worked" from "Who Will Benefit From Psychotherapy?" (Pg. 69) by Lester E. Luborsky, Ph.D.

Chapter 19

Treatment Facilities for the Severely Depressed

Only a small minority who are extremely depressed (e.g., with a history of suicide attempts or a failure to improve with outpatient therapy) require hospitalization. The vast majority can receive very effective treatment just by visiting a psychiatrist or mental health professional on an occasional basis at his (her) office without disruption to their lives.

For those unfortunate few, the following is a description of the main types of treatment centers:

1. Major medical centers. Often linked to medical schools, these prestigious organizations provide both inpatient and outpatient facilities for a comprehensive range of mental illnesses. Backed by leading specialists in the field and well funded research departments, they are particularly well suited to diagnose and treat depression which does not respond to the usual types of treatment. More staff is usually available than in both private and public psychiatric hospitals.

   Some offer free programs offering new types of treatment in exchange for assisting in their research. These are almost always well supervised with rigorous and frequent check-ups and therefore good value. The centers are also an excellent source of referral and information.

2. Private psychiatric hospitals. Offering greater privacy and a more pleasant environment than public hospitals, private psychiatric hospitals tend to specialize in short-term care lasting less than six months. Treatment is usually geared towards each individual's needs, and more staff are made available to attend to each patient.

Some private hospitals specialize in specific disorders (e.g., phobic depressions) or types of patient (e.g., children or the elderly). Because fees, insurance coverage and standard of care naturally vary between institutions, careful inquiries should be made by prospective patients. (There have been some recent scandals concerning private hospitals.) Approval by the Joint Commission of Accreditation of Hospitals is a must; this means that an institution meets a basic standard of care.

3. Community hospitals. Many hospitals in small communities place all patients together in the general wards. Only some offer doctors and staff on a full-time basis, while others contract them to work only a few hours each day or week. This is probably not the best option for a patient with severe depression. (It could be suitable for a mildly depressed person; but then such a person is better off seeking outpatient treatment.)

4. Publicly funded hospitals. All states and large cities provide free (or low cost) services for the impoverished, including long-term inpatient treatment. However, the facilities and personal attention are not as good as those of private institutions owing to funding and staffing problems.

   Former military personnel are also eligible for help from Veterans Administration (VA) hospitals which are funded by the government.

5. Freestanding mental health clinics. Basing their fees on ability to pay, these are a better solution for those who find it difficult to pay. Many receive grants from the government and are run by a group of mental health professionals, a hospital or local health agency. Standards are variable and should be checked before treatment.

6. Emergency care. All major hospitals contain emergency rooms, e.g., for a severely depressed patient who has just attempted suicide and might do so again. Treatment is usually free but some private hospitals may attempt to divert patients without insurance. Standards of care vary and waiting times are often long.

A relative or friend who is concerned for someone who may be in such a danger would be advised to check out the local emergency facilities in advance.

7. Partial care. Offered by some hospitals and freestanding clinics, this is an intermediate step between full time hospitalization and occasional out-patient treatment. The patient usually attends only during the daytime, thus saving expensive overnight stays. A full range of short-term, intensive treatments is provided, including individual, group and family therapy.

©BRILLIANT ENTERPRISES 1976
POT-SHOTS NO. 908
SORRY
I WANT
A SIGNED
APOLOGY
FROM THE WORLD,
FOR THE WAY
IT HAS BEEN TREATING ME.
Ashleigh Brilliant

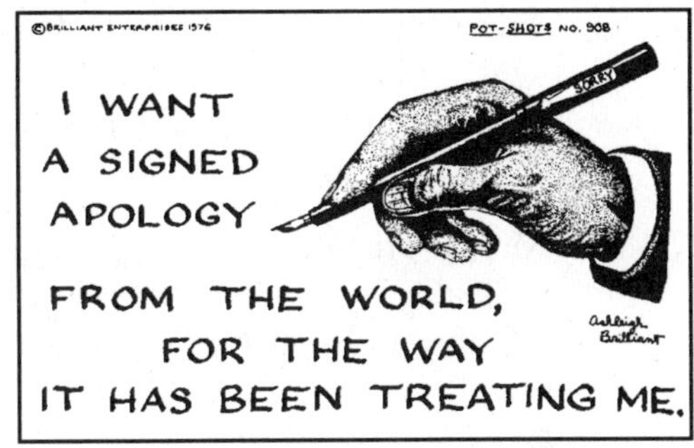

8. Sheltered residential care. This is ideal for the severely depressed who do not require hospitalization but are not yet able to function on their own. While treatment proceeds, the patient can build up his (her) life with the aim of eventual independence. It is an excellent way to build up confidence and self-dignity in the early stages of recovery, when mental concentration is poor, self-esteem is low, and vulnerability is high. Job rehabilitation may be available.

   Often called a "halfway house," sheltered residential care is similar to sheltered accommodation for the elderly, providing amenities such as meals, laundry, recreational facilities, and ready access to medical treatment when needed. A manager or member of staff provides supervision and emotional support.

A good mental health treatment center is best found by seeking a recommendation from a psychiatrist or mental health practitioner who is familiar with the local treatment facilities. Mental health support and advocacy groups are also a good source of information, paticularly the National Alliance for the Mentally Ill (NAMI) and the National Depressive and Manic-Depressive Association (NDMDA). (Look under the list of self-help organizations in the References and Sources (page 243).) Alternatively, a list of hospitals and care centers can be obtained from one of the following manuals in the local library:

1. "The American Hospital Association Guide to the Health Care Field" published by the American Hospital Association, 1 North Franklin Street, Chicago, IL 60606 (tel. 800-242-2626 or 312-422-3000).

2. "Mental Health Directory" published by the U.S. Department of Health and Human Services (Institute of Mental Health), available through the Superintendent of Documents, Government Printing Office, P.O. Box 371954, Pittsburgh, PA 15250 (tel. 202-512-1800).

Courage is not freedom from fear; it is being afraid and carrying on.

Anonymous

Chapter 20

Cost of Treatment

Medical fees for the treatment of depression vary greatly, depending on the practitioner. As mentioned elsewhere, higher charges do not necessarily mean better treatment. An annual survey of fees is conducted by "Psychotherapy Finances" (a newsletter published by Ridgewood Financial Institute, Inc.). According to the 1995 survey, fees have risen only very gradually over the last three years at a rate of approximately 2% per annum.

Mental health professionals will quote you their "usual and customary" fee. This is what they charge to individuals who contact them directly and are not covered by insurance. If someone claims hardship (e.g., recent loss of a job), some professionals may be willing to reduce their fee on a "sliding scale" according to the patient's means. Practitioners with a light workload are likely to do so; those who are very busy are not.

Treatment sessions are normally 45 or 50 minutes long. Typical "usual and customary" fees per session are as follows:

FEES FOR SOLO PRACTITIONERS

Type of practitioner	Usual fee per session ($)
Psychiatrist	100–130
Psychologist	90–100
Social worker	70–85
Marriage and family therapist	75–90
Professional counselor	70–85

Rates are fairly uniform across the United States. It should be borne in mind that the fee ranges above are only typical, with some practitioners charging substantially more and some substantially less. Some local areas are traditionally more expensive, e.g. Manhattan, New York. On the other hand, rural practitioners may charge a little less.

A well-informed source at the National Depressive and Manic-Depressive Association (NDMDA) (who requested anonymity) has found that many practitioners in university towns with psychiatric departments charge rates $25–50 per session higher than in neighboring towns although the standard of their treatment is no higher. The conclusion for those who wish to save money is obvious.

About 40% of practices are run as a group of two, three, four, or more mental health practitioners. Group practices charge much less than solo practitioners; their typical "usual and customary" fees per session are as follows:

FEES FOR GROUP PRACTITIONERS

Type of practitioner	Usual fee per session ($)
Psychiatrist	50–70
Psychologist	40–50
Social worker	35–45
Marriage and family therapist	25–40
Professional counselor	30–45

It is common for psychologists and social workers (who provide therapy) to liaise with psychiatrists (who prescribe medications). This allows each of these to specialize in what they are best at. In addition, this arrangement helps keep down fees.

Medications vary in cost, with drugs available in generic form cheaper than the brand name equivalents. Obviously, the more medications required, the higher the cost. Typically, one can expect to spend twenty cents to two dollars per day.

Most people are members of health insurance plans directly or through their employers. A growing trend is for insurance companies and employers to contract with an intermediary "managed-care company" to arrange and supervise health care for their clients. Employers, insurance companies, and managed care companies negotiate with mental (and other) health professionals in order to pay reduced fees. In practice, the reduction amounts to 15–20%.

Some employers and insurance companies agree a "capitation fee" (e.g., $5 per month per employee/insured person to cover all claims and treatment needs) with the managed-care companies. In turn, the latter occasionally arrange the same (at a lower rate) with a number of mental (and other) health professionals. Unfortunately, such arrangements may encourage limited treatment although managed-care plans are supposed to provide as much treatment as is necessary.

Traditional insurance companies (who pay practitioners' fees directly) tend to put limits on the number of treatment sessions they are willing to pay for. In addition, they normally pay only a percentage of the fee up to a specified maximum.

Managed-care companies are very cost-conscious and look for practitioners who can show that their treatment is effective in terms of quality, time and cost. As a result, more and more practitioners are providing "outcomes research," collected from patients by means of brief surveys. At present, only 20% of practitioners collect any data which, in the author's opinion, is essential for the patient in order to track recovery. Nevertheless, this is an improvement on the past since traditionally practitioners did no monitoring at all.

In turn, employers and insurance companies are demanding "outcomes research" from managed-care companies in order to assess their performance.

According to Herbert E. Klein, editor and publisher of "Psychotherapy Finances," the usual forms of psychotherapy given are interpersonal, behavior, and cognitive-behavior therapy. In practice, providing a mixture of therapies is popular among mental health professionals. Their treatment is "symptom based," namely, geared to whatever works best and quickest for the patient.

Because of cost pressures, time-limited therapies are most common. The normal number of sessions are between 10 and 25. Psychoanalysis, which tends to require many months and often years of intensive treatment, is hardly ever given except to "rich actors and millionaires" (sic) who can afford it.

> *It does not take much strength to do things, but it requires great strength to decide on what to do.*
>
> Anonymous

Chapter 21

Sources of Free or Cheap Help .... No Reason Why You Have to Spend a Fortune Getting Treatment

Matthew Lesko, author of "What to Do When You Can't Afford Health Care," conducted a survey where one hundred cardiologists were approached about examining a woman who could not afford to pay. The woman had been prescribed an anti-depressant drug and her doctor said she needed a simple heart examination before she could take it. The cardiologists' replies were as follows:

Agreed to examine for free without money or insurance	4%
Would not examine but gave helpful suggestions	5%
Refused to examine, gave unhelpful suggestions and/or could not give any advice	91%
Total	100%

Assuming this is true of all doctors, this means that more than nine out of ten have no idea where to turn to when you do not have health insurance. In fact, help and treatment is available and this section explains how to get it.

1. Treatment by an NIH Clinical Center

Free treatment can be obtained by joining a clinical trial funded by private drug companies or the federal government. First of all, try the National Institutes of Health (NIH) Clinical Center. The NIH is a health research institution funded by the federal government. Its clinical center contains a hospital with over 400 beds for inpatient treatment. Outpatients are catered for at the adjacent Ambulatory Care Research Facility. The Patient Referral Line (tel. 301-496-4891) will let you know whether your condition is being studied, the name of the primary investigator, and whether you meet the requirements for the study.

For more information, write to the Clinical Center, National Institutes of Health, 9000 Rockville Pike, Bethesda, MD 20892 (tel. 301-496-2563). (See later for information on individual institutes.)

The Clinical Center at Bethesda admits approximately 9,600 patients for hospital care and handles more than 85,000 visits at its outpatient clinics. All this is federally funded in the name of research. It is not only the lucky and rich who benefit. However, the chances are that your doctor will not be aware of this program so you will need to bring it to his (her) attention.

The Clinical Center cooperates fully with referring doctors and psychiatrists, who submit a diagnosis and medical history. A full report is made available after the end of the course of treatment. Sometimes follow-up observations are requested from the patient's doctor in his (her) home city.

All medical and hospital services are free; all the patient has to pay for is transportation. In cases of emergency and/or extreme hardship, assistance may be obtained from the Clinical Center Social Work Department (tel. 301-496-2381).

In order to qualify for treatment by the NIH you must satisfy four requirements:

(a) Your doctor must refer you. The referral should include:
 (1) your current psychiatric diagnosis (Axes I and II on the DSM-IV scale)
 (2) a summary of the course of your illness
 (3) treatments received and the response
 (4) discharge summaries of all psychiatric hospitalizations during the last five years
 (5) a statement of your physical health
 (6) history of alcohol and substance abuse (if applicable)

(b) Your type of depression must be under current investigation.

(c) You must satisfy certain age, weight, sex and general health requirements.

(d) You have to understand what it means and voluntarily consent to participate in a research study.

A current "index of studies" (updated quarterly) is available on the AMA/GTE Telenet Medical Information Network.

The place most like to have a research study on depression is the National Institute of Mental Health (NIMH). Your doctor or you should make inquiries here first. For contact names, addresses and telephone numbers, and a list of Clinical studies conducted in 1996 on depression (and areas related to depression), see References and Sources (page 189).

Other national institutes occasionally conduct studies related to depression and may be worth a call. They are the:

(a) National Institute on Aging (NIA)
(b) National Institute on Alcohol Abuse and Alcoholism (NIAAA)
(c) National Institute on Child Health and Human Development (NICHHD)
(d) National Institute on Drug Abuse (NIDA)

For contact names, addresses and telephone numbers, see References and Sources (page 190).

> *The harder you work, the luckier you get.*
>
> Gay Player (1935–)

2. Treatment from Doctors Who Receive Grants to Study Your Illness

Thousands of doctors throughout the United States receive research money and may be able to treat your illness free of charge. The National Institutes of Health (Division of Research Grants) can help you locate one of these doctors by searching a computer database named CRISP (Computer Retrieval for Information on Scientific Projects). This search, conducted free of charge, will provide you with the study title, researcher, organization, grant amount, and detailed description of the research project. Contact: The Division of Research Grants, National Institutes of Health, 6701 Rockledge Drive, MSC 7762, Suite 3032, Bethesda, MD 20892 (tel. 301-435-0714).

When you have this list, ask your doctor to refer you to the project contact.

Keep in mind that you may be placed in a study where you are given a placebo. Although this is a risk, many research programs offer to give a few months of free treatment with an effective drug once you are off the study.

For a list of institutions funded by the National Institutes of Health in 1996 to conduct projects related to depression, see under References and Sources (page 191).

3. Free Health Care at Your Hospital

Many hospitals provide free or low-cost health care to those who are on low incomes. Usually this is done under what is called the Hill-Burton free care program. To apply for this type of assistance, you have to show that your income satisfies the Poverty Income Guidelines.

Every Hill-Burton facility has to provide a certain amount of care every year at reduced cost or free of charge. However, it has the right to choose what kind of treatment and services this covers. On request it will provide you with a list (called the "Individual Notice") describing what is covered in detail. Even if you do not qualify for this program, a facility may have special funds to help you anyway.

Hospital business offices will help you apply for government assistance and set up payment plans within your budget.

For information on the Hill-Burton program, including eligibility requirements, facilities required to provide assistance in your area, and complaint procedures, contact: The Bureau of Health Resources Development, Health Resources and Services Administration, Department of Health and Human Services, 5600 Fishers Lane, Room 7-31, Rockville, MD 20857 (tel. 800-638-0742 outside MD and 800-492-0359 inside MD).

Ask for a list of facilities sorted in city order within your state. When you receive it, call up the facilities near you and ask them for their Individual Notice under the Hill-Burton Program.

4. Local Free Health Clinics

Many local health department provide clinics which charge nothing or according to a sliding-fee scale. These clinics and screening centers cater for non-emergency situations, e.g., depression. Services and charges vary from area to area. According to the National Association of Community Health Centers, as many as ten to twelve million people benefit from these clinics which are sponsored by the federal and local governments.

Demand is very strong is some areas for the services that these clinics provide and there may be long waiting lists. Check this out by contacting your local health department. You can find the address and telephone number either by looking in the blue pages of your phone book or by contacting your local State Department of Public Health. (See References and Sources (page 199).)

©ASHLEIGH BRILLIANT 1983.
POT-SHOTS NO. 2952
Ashleigh Brilliant
I'M THINKING OF QUITTING ALL MY ACTIVITIES,
IN ORDER TO DEVOTE FULL-TIME TO MY BOREDOM.

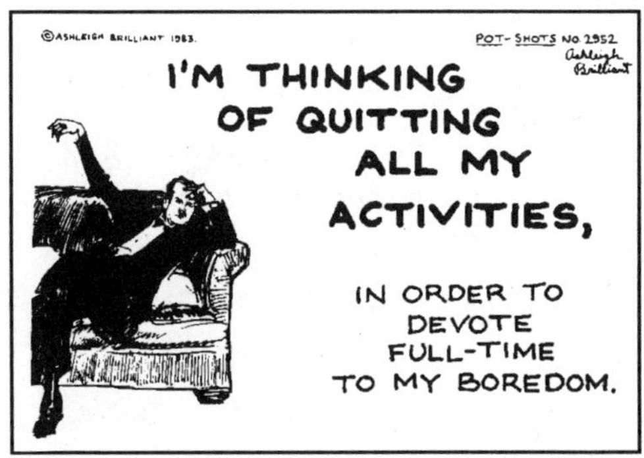

5. Federal and State Medical Programs

The federal government funds programs to support the health needs of senior citizens, the disabled and those on low incomes. Medicare is a federal health insurance program which funds those who are more than 65 years old and those with certain disabilities.

Medicaid, a joint federal and state program, funds the health needs of the indigent and the "medically needy." Conditions of eligibility, and facilities and services offered vary from state to state. These can be ascertained by contacting your local Medicare/Medicaid office health department.

You can find the address and telephone number of your nearest office by looking in the blue pages of your phone book (under Human Services). Alternatively, you may contact: Medicare Hotline, Healthcare Financing Administration, 7500 Security Boulevard, Baltimore, MD 21244 (tel. 800-638-6833). This hotline will give information and booklets about Medicare. The Medicaid hotline is situated at the same address (tel. 410-786-7144).

6. Free Health care for Children, Adolescents and Pregnant Mothers

Grants (called "Title V" block) are given by the federal government to each state to provide maternal, child and adolescent health care. The funds are handed over to the Maternal and Child Health Division of the state Department of Health. 30% has to be allocated to children with special health care needs and 30% to children and adolescents. The allocation of the remaining 40% is left to the discretion of each state.

All states are required by federal law to provide Medicaid to pregnant women and children up to the age of six inclusive whose income is no more than one third above the poverty line. (This is approximately $7,000 for one person, $9,500 for two, $12,000 for three and $14,500 for four people. Many states provide additional benefits.

More information can be found by contacting the local department of health, whose address and telephone number can be found in the blue pages of your phone book. Another source of information is the Maternal and Child Health Care Division of the state Department of Health, which usually has a free "800" telephone number. (See References and Sources (page 207).)

Persistent people begin their success where others end in failure.
Anonymous

7. Getting Prescription Drugs Free of Charge

Getting prescribed drugs is vital for the severely depressed, many of whom are too ill to work or hold down a job. In fact, for the suicidally inclined, it is literally a matter of life and death. Unfortunately, many simply cannot afford to buy them. Therefore, they cannot recover and get a job where they could afford to pay. If this is you or someone you know, this section explains how to get out of this vicious circle.

Unknown to most people, many drug companies do have programs offering prescription drugs free of charge to people just like yourself. Eligibility requirements vary from manufacturer to manufacturer. For example, you may need to show proof of limited income, declare a lack of insurance coverage, or provide a doctor's referral.

Most companies send the drugs (and refills) directly to your doctor. Sometimes there are delays before you can receive them so check the procedure with the manufacturer beforehand.

The "Directory of Prescription Drug Patient Assistance Programs," published by the Pharmaceutical Research and Manufacturers of America (PhRMA), details the programs and conditions of individual drug manufacturers. For further information, contact: Pharmaceutical Research and Manufacturers of America, located at 1100 15 Street, NW, Washington, DC 20005, (tel. 800-PMA-INFO). A list of companies which manufacture drugs that combat depression, requirements for obtaining free prescription drugs, and whom to contact is printed in the References and Sources (see page 217).

8. Free Treatment at Hospital Emergency Rooms

By federal law, hospital emergency rooms are required to assess a patient's condition through a preliminary screening. Also, they must treat and stabilize all emergency situations. This is useful for anyone whose depression is so severe that he (she) feels suicidal.

Hospitals have the right to charge for emergency treatment. In practice, however, an indigent patient who cannot afford to pay will end up getting the treatment for nothing.

Emergency medicine covers taking immediate action to prevent death and any further disability in a health crisis, stabilizing the condition of the patient, and making a short-term assessment beyond the immediate threat to life and limb.

If you know of someone who is denied treatment in this way, you can complain to the regional Health Care Financing Administration (of the U.S. Department of Health and Human Services) who will take up the matter. Unfortunately, a person who is severely depressed is unlikely to be in a position to make a complaint owing to his (her) poor state of health. Therefore, if you are severely depressed and decide to go to the hospital emergency room, try and persuade a relative or friend to accompany you and make sure you get the treatment you deserve.

It is best to use this service as a last resort because emergency waiting rooms tend to be crowded and waiting times may be very long. Incidentally, if you are depressed and on low income, do not wait until you are so severely ill that you need to visit the hospital emergency room! (This may sound ridiculous; some people really do that.) Use the other free or cheap options described here and get better as soon as possible. Above all, do not delay and let yourself suffer.

A list of regional Health Care Financing Administration offices is shown in References and Sources (page 223).

> *It takes as much courage to try and fail as it does to try and succeed.*
>
> Anonymous

9. Local Volunteer Doctors

Many doctors give some of their time for free or at a reduced charge. On average this comes to 6.6 hours per week per physician, according to a survey conducted by the American Medical Association (AMA), amounting to an overall $6.8 billion of services every year.

Details of local services, which vary from area to area, can be obtained from your State Medical Association whose addresses and telephone numbers are listed in References and Sources (page 227).

10. Free Information and Advice

Free information and advice about depression is available from Project D/ART (Depression/Awareness, Recognition, Treatment), a major media campaign run by the National Institute of Mental Health (NIMH) in collaboration with other organizations. D/ART publishes many booklets and reports; topics include recognizing symptoms, causes, treatments, and latest research. (Many are also available in Spanish.) These can be requested from: The National Institute of Mental Health, 5600 Fishers Lane, Room 7C02, Rockville, MD 20857 (tel. 301-443-4515).

Information specific to depression and the elderly can also be obtained from: The National Institute on Aging, Building 31, Room 5C27, Bethesda, MD 20892 (tel. 301-496-1752).

Free (or cheap) publications including a brief description of the contents are printed in the References and Sources (see page 233). A summary of the titles is as follows:

FREE (OR CHEAP) PUBLICATIONS	
From the National Institute of Mental Health:	
General publications:	
1.	A Consumer's Guide to Mental Health Services
2.	Bipolar Disorder
3.	D/ART Fact Sheet
4.	Depression: Patients Get Younger as Rx Options Increase
5.	Depression: What You Need to Know
6.	Depression: Effective Treatments are Available
7.	Depressive Illnesses: Treatments Bring New Hope
8.	Helpful Facts About Depressive Disorders
9.	Helping the Depressed Person Get Treatment
10.	If You're Over 65 and Feeling Depressed ... Treatment Brings New Hope
11.	Information About D/ART and Depression

FREE (OR CHEAP) PUBLICATIONS

From the National Institute of Mental Health:

12. Let's Talk About Depression

13. Plain Talk About Depression

14. Plain Talk About Handling Stress

15. What to Do When a Friend is Depressed: A Guide for Students

16. You Are Not Alone

Publications for the workplace:

17. The Mentally Restored and Work: A Successful Partnership

18. Eight Questions Employers Ask About Hiring the Mentally Restored

19. Managing Depression in the Workplace

20. Poster for Employers: "Not Everyone With Depression Is This Visible"

21. What to Do When an Employee is Depressed: A Guide for Supervisors

Publications of professional interest:

22. Approaching the 21st Century: Opportunities for NIMH Neuroscience Research 1988

23. ECA Update

24. National Plan for Research on Child and Adolescent Mental Disorders

25. Psychopharmacology Bulletin (Quarterly Journal)

26. Suicide Facts

27. The Value of Psychiatric Treatment: Its Efficacy in Severe Mental Disorders

FREE (OR CHEAP) PUBLICATIONS

From the National Institute of Mental Health:

Publications in Spanish:

28. Datos Utiles Sobre Enfermedadas Depresivas

29. Depresion/Advertencia, Reconocimiento, Tratamiento

30. Depresion: Lo Que Usted Necesita Saber

31. La Depresion: Existen Tratamientos Eficaces

32. No Estas Solo: Datos Acerca de Salud Mental y Enfermedades

33. Platica Franca Sobre La Tension

34. Una Guia Sobre Servicios De Salud Mental Para Los Consumidores

From the National Institute on Aging:

35. Diagnosis and Treatment of Depression in Late Life

36. Perspectives in Health Promotion and Aging (Quarterly Journal)

37. Fact Sheet: How Physical and Mental Health Interact in Older Persons

38. Fact Sheet: Mental Health and Aging; Scientific Discoveries and Prospects

39. Fact Sheet: Depression in the Elderly

Videos, tapes, computer software, and other audiovisuals about depression can be obtained from your local library by means of an interlibrary loan from: The National Library of Medicine, 8600 Rockville Pike, Bethesda, MD 20894 (tel. 800-272-4787). For full details of titles and brief descriptions, see References and Sources (page 238).

Titles, for which there may be a nominal charge, include:

AUDIOVISUALS	
From the National Library of Medicine:	
Video recordings:	
40.	Downtime: Understanding Clinical Depression in the Worksite
41.	Overcoming Depression
42.	Treating Depression: Preventing Suicide
43.	Treating Depression in the Elderly
44.	Diagnosis and Treatment of Anxiety and Depression in the Elderly
45.	Newer Treatments for Depression
46.	Reducing Resident Depression: Assessment and Intervention
47.	Teen and Childhood Depression
48.	Women and Disease
49.	Atypical Depression
50.	Depression: New Treatment Options
51.	Depression: The Storm Within
52.	Depression
53.	What About Prozac?
54.	Crying for Happiness
55.	Depression and the Elderly
56.	ECT in the Treatment of Major Depression
57.	Geriatric Psychopharmacology: An Update
58.	Management of Depression in Childhood
59.	Psychotherapy of Depression
60.	Coping with Aging
61.	Diagnosis of Depression in Adolescents
62.	Manic Depression: The Agony and The Ecstacy
63.	Teen Suicide and Depression

AUDIOVISUALS

From the National Library of Medicine:

Cassette tape recordings:

64.	Panic Disorder, Agoraphobia, and Depression
65.	Depression and Suicide: Multidisciplinary Assessment and Treatment
66.	Manic Depression: Voices of an Illness
67.	Maternal Depression and Early Child Development
68.	Mood Altering Agents
69.	Postpartum Depression: Therapeutic Teamwork Between Psychiatry and Pediatrics
70.	Postpartum Depression: Research and Clinical Perspectives
71.	Special Problems in the Psychotherapy of Depression
72.	Depression: Diagnosis and Treatment
73.	Depression in Childhood and Adolescence

Happiness lies in the joy of achievement and the thrill of creative effort.

Franklin D. Roosevelt (1882–1945)

PART THREE:

OVERCOMING DEPRESSION

Chapter 22

Depression in Childhood and Adolescence

Many adults say that they spent the best part of their lives in childhood. While for most children this period is a carefree and happy time, for a sizeable minority (about 15–20%) it is a very miserable and difficult experience.

Depression strikes not only at adults, but also at children and adolescents. Unlike adults, children often react to depression by being restless, irritable, disruptive, behaving badly, and breaking into tantrums. Performance at school goes down. Many have difficulty in concentrating or fall into daydreams; many get into trouble and become unpopular with the staff and other children try to avoid them. Others become very shy and find it difficult to make friends. Some fall victim to bullies.

POT-SHOTS NO. 4389.
THE FUTURE SEEMS TO BE IN GOOD HANDS~
IT'S THE PAST I'M WORRIED ABOUT.
Ashleigh Brilliant
©ASHLEIGH BRILLIANT 1988.

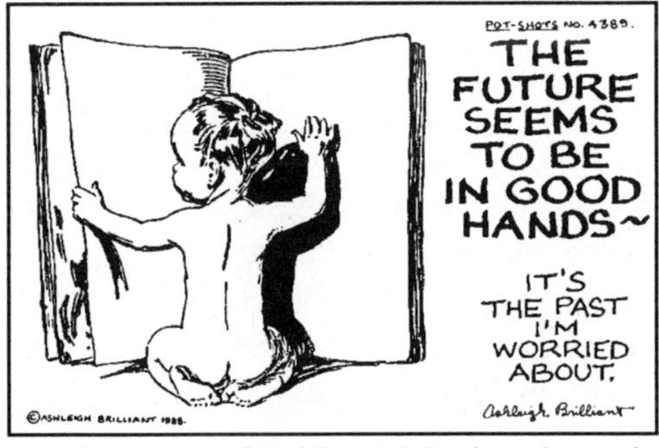

Only a few decades ago, it was thought that depression affected only adults. If children showed symptoms, it was regarded as a passing phase of their development. However, this is not the case. As mentioned in a previous chapter, proneness to depression tends to be hereditary in some families. Maybe there is something in a person's gene structure that causes him (her) to react extremely badly to upsets and disappointments, or slide into depression for apparently no reason at all.

Many people who suffer from severe or recurrent depression (and manic depression, i.e., depressions alternating with manic episodes) in their adulthood can trace the roots to their childhood or adolescence. It is best to treat the illness as early as possible, at the time of onset, before it gets out of hand. Another good reason is because these are the people who mostly respond best to medication. Once recovered, they need never suffer again. They can either take a regular maintenance dose of medicine or take the medicine again immediately when they detect the illness coming on again.

Never again need they live with a cloud over their heads: the risk of poor assertiveness, being bullied, finding themselves unable to hold down a job, attacks of lethargy, withdrawal from social life, losing friends, coping badly with domestic responsibilities, etc. In other words, they can live the rest of their lives in the confidence of social fulfillment, career success, domestic happiness, etc.

Adolescents are particularly at risk of depression because they are going through a period of fundamental emotional development, determining their identity as they grow into mature adults. A disruption to this process can leave emotional scars that may take many years to pass.

> *Children are like sponges. They absorb all your strength and leave you limp. But give them a squeeze and you get it all back.*
>
> Anonymous

One reads too many tales in the newspapers nowadays of promising youngsters who have committed suicide by taking an overdose of drugs or by some other distressing method. People who knew them often remark they did not have a clue that they were so depressed, except that the youngsters used to complain about being bullied incessantly and cruelly. Often these children were very bright academically. Their parents grieve while their teachers scratch their heads in despair. Everyone feels helpless.

The author believes that there should be widespread screening programs at schools for depression in order to eradicate most instances of this scourge when it first appears and before it gets worse. A few such programs have already been implemented.

Meanwhile, parents with relatives who have suffered from depression (or manic depression) in the past, even long in the past, would be wise to have their children screened for this illness regularly, for example every year. This could be part of a general health checkup.

Below is a list of typical symptoms of childhood depression. In most cases these symptoms reflect a marked change in a child's usual pattern of behavior and are prolonged, lasting more than about two weeks. It is usual for a depressed child to exhibit most but not all of these symptoms. For example, there are many depressed children who are very withdrawn and not aggressive at all.

TYPICAL SYMPTOMS OF CHILDHOOD DEPRESSION

1.	Sadness
2.	Quietness
3.	Loneliness
4.	Lethargy
5.	Complaints of boredom
6.	Bad sleeping habits; too much or too little sleep
7.	Lack of appetite
8.	Poor physical growth due to poor nutrition
9.	Slow development
10.	Favorite target for bullies
11.	Difficulty making friends; few if any friends
12.	Problems at school: **(a)** poor concentration **(b)** daydreaming **(c)** lack of interest **(d)** disruptive behavior (sometimes) **(e)** exam failures **(f)** drop in grades
13.	Low self-esteem; feeling guilty, "dumb," stupid
14.	Irritability
15.	Aggressive behavior
16.	Suicidal thoughts (often not noticed or ignored)

Adolescent depression may be set off by events that adults (including parents) may think trivial or exaggerated. Nevertheless, adults should appreciate that teenagers see things differently for themselves. These events include arguments with parents; e.g., over how late they may stay out of the house, disciplinary problems, the break up of a romantic relationship, failing a mid-term examination, rapid or slow physical growth in comparison with peers, and even the appearance of acne or pimples on the face.

A healthy teenager will get over these disappointments in a few days or weeks at the most. If grieving or moping goes on for much longer, it is a sign that treatment should be started. Not only the teenager suffers; so do his (her) parents and family. The problem should be resolved as soon as possible.

ADDITIONAL TYPICAL SYMPTOMS OF ADOLESCENT DEPRESSION	
1.	Increased social withdrawal
2.	Little interest and pleasure in many activities previously enjoyed
3.	Extreme dietary fads
4.	Neglect of grooming and personal appearance
5.	Preoccupation with death
6.	Drugs and/or alcohol abuse
7.	Feeling of failure
8.	Little interest in planning for the future

Providing treatment

Diagnosis and treatment should be put into the hands of a psychiatrist who specializes in children and adolescents, and can distinguish between depression and normal development. He (she) will have a special approach in dealing with them in order to talk at their level and gain their confidence. Naturally, this requires a great deal of skill. Ideally, the practitioner will have had qualified training and at least two years experience working full time with children, and be certified by the American Board of Psychiatry and Neurology (ABPN).

Besides finding out information from the youngster about his (her) problems, the psychiatrist should want to talk to the parents and get opinions from the teachers in school. Often medication and/or therapy bring rapid beneficial results to the delight of everyone concerned. Although medication may be given at a different level than for adults, the side effects tend to be weaker and shorter lasting.

Because the youngster usually lives in a family setting, therapy may directly or indirectly involve the parents, brothers, sisters, and other relatives. They need to understand what he (she) is going through and appreciate that their behavior affects the behavior and well-being of the youngster and vice versa.

YOUTHFUL SUICIDES

Suicide at a young age is more common than most people think. Did you know that:

1. Suicide is the third leading cause of death after traffic accidents and homicides for older teenagers.
2. 7,000 teenagers kill themselves every year, and 400,000 attempt suicide.
3. Five- and six-year-olds have tried to kill themselves (the lowest documented age is 2½ years).
4. Half of youth suicides result from depression (estimate).
5. Youth suicides have tripled in the last thirty years.

Modern psychology tells us that it's bad to be an orphan, terrible to be an only child, damaging to be the youngest, crushing to be in the middle, and taxing to be the oldest. There seems to be no way out, except to be born an adult.

Anonymous

Chapter 23

Depression in the Elderly

As doctors discover more ways to cure serious illnesses, and medicines become more effective, people are living longer and longer. The proportion of senior citizens in the population is increasing year by year. At present it is approximately 12%, that is over 30 million people. It is estimated that 15–20% of them, about 5 million senior citizens, suffer from depression.

Unfortunately, the illness is often misdiagnosed as incurable senile dementia, leaving hundreds of thousands to suffer miserably and unnecessarily.

Events which may trigger depression in the elderly include job retirement, reduced income, consequent restructuring of life routines, loss of a spouse and friends, moving to a nursing home, moving away from friends, and feeling superfluous and unimportant.

©ASHLEIGH BRILLIANT 1988
POT-SHOTS NO. 4588
GETTING OLDER
IS NOT SO BAD,
IF YOU
DO IT WITH
SOMEONE
YOU LOVE.
Ashleigh Brilliant

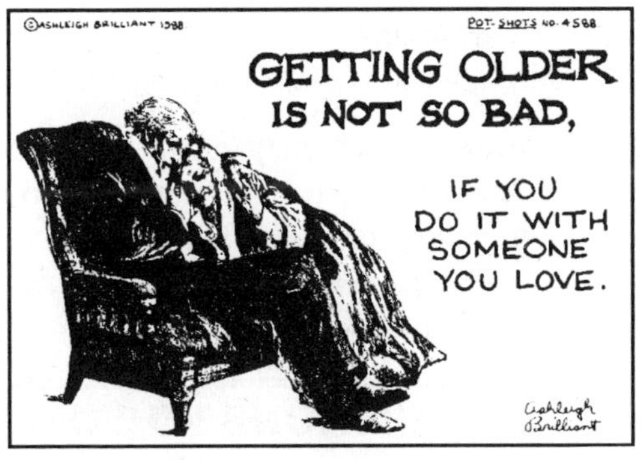

Housebound people living alone and depending on a home attendant have every reason to fall into depression.

Nursing homes, many of which lack a stimulating atmosphere and where the residents feel isolated and lonely, are a big cause of depression. This is intensified when relatives and friends are reluctant to visit. As many as one quarter of the residents of a poorly run nursing home may be severely depressed. Anyone who has visited one of these institutions and seen the glum faces, vacant stares and lethargic behavior will understand why.

Depression saps away the will to live and it is not surprising that depressed elderly people tend to die earlier than those who are not. Moreover, the rate of suicide among the elderly is twice that of the rest of the population.

> *Old age is like flying a plane through a storm. Once you're aboard, there's nothing you can do.*
>
> Golda Meir (1898–1978)

Depression may also come about through certain illnesses such as:

1. hypertension (high blood pressure)
2. hyper- and hypothyroidism
3. Cushing's disease
4. Parkinson's disease
5. strokes
6. heart complaints
7. lung disorders
8. carcinoma
9. Alzheimer's disease

Medications which may cause depression in the elderly are mainly those used to treat hypertension and Parkinson's disease. Some hormone medicines also fall into this category. Frequently, depression arises from taking a large number of medications which are appropriate individually but not in combination. The list includes:

MEDICATIONS WHICH CAN TRIGGER OFF DEPRESSION

	Generic Name	Brand name
	For hypertension:	
1.	Clonidine	Catapres
2.	Hydralazine	Apresoline Hydrochloride
3.	Methyldopa	Aldomet
4.	Propranolol	Inderal
5.	Reserpine	Serpasil, Ser-Ap-Es, Sandril

MEDICATIONS WHICH CAN TRIGGER OFF DEPRESSION		
Generic Name		**Brand name**
	For Parkinson's disease:	
6.	Levodopa	Dopar, Larodopa
7.	Levodopa and carbidopa	Sinemet
8.	Bromocriptine	
	Hormones	
9.	Estrogen	
10.	Progesterone	
11.	Cortisone	
12.	Prednisone	

Providing treatment

Just as with children and adolescents, it is advantageous to be diagnosed and treated by a practitioner who has already gained a lot of experience with the elderly. Besides talking to the patient, the doctor who is making a diagnosis will need to be made aware of all medications currently being taken.

Elderly people who are ill with depression may appear to be confused and agitated, and exhibit a loss of memory. Depression often mimics dementia and other brain dysfunctions, and the trained and sensitive doctor will be able to distinguish one from the other. Tests may include an electroencephalogram (EEG), a computerized axial tomogram of the brain (CAT scan), thyroid function studies and blood analysis.

Dementia is sometimes combined with depression which is not recognized. However, when the depression is treated, the dementia usually subsides.

Results which show no physical cause for the depressed mood will indicate depression, especially if there is a family history of depression. Treatment can clear up the symptoms remarkably within a few months and the patient become much brighter and happier. In many cases, instead of having to enter a nursing home, the formerly depressed senior citizen can enjoy a fulfilled and self-sufficient life.

When medication is decided upon, the doctor has to take care that it does not interfere detrimentally with drugs already being administered. Side effects, in particular, must be watched carefully. Blood pressure and urine samples need to be checked regularly until the therapeutic level is reached. Doses tend to be less than for younger adults; typically one third to one half the normal dose. Since more time is required for the medication to become effective, dosages should not be increased too soon in order to prevent overmedication of the patient.

Newer antidepressants, including selective serotonin reuptake inhibitors (SSRIs) (e.g., Prozac and Zoloft), are the favorites of physicians because of their effectiveness and the relatively mild side effects, especially when started in low doses. However, some tricyclic antidepressants (e.g., Pamelor and Norpramin) may be preferred because they stimulate appetite (unlike Prozac and Zoloft). On the other hand, other drugs (e.g., Elavil, Sinequan, Surmontil and Vivactil) are avoided because they frequently cause confusion as a side effect.

Patients with poor heart conditions may best be treated with electroconvulsive therapy (ECT). Contrary to popular belief, this method has not only the fewest side effects, but also is usually the safest and most effective method of treatment for those with severe depression.

According to a recent report in the "American Journal of Psychiatry" (November 1994), German scientists have discovered that depression may cause osteoporosis (thinning of the bones) through hormonal changes. Therefore, it is a good idea to add a daily calcium supplement to the treatment.

> *You know you're old when you discover that your children are learning in history class what you studied in current events.*
>
> Anonymous

Chapter 24

Depression in Women

Men can read this chapter, too! Traditionally, women have been looked upon as more vulnerable then men. Men traditionally play the fighting and dominant roles; women the submissive and homemaking roles. Men are supposed to be able to show a "stiff upper lip" while women will burst into tears in times of crisis.

These traditional roles extend into the realms of emotional health. On the one hand, women can be expected to cry and be depressed from time to time. On the other hand, men are expected never to show depression and the exceptional ones who do are regarded as "weaklings."

This "tradition" is nothing more than a myth. Fortunately, with the equalization of men's and women's roles, it is becoming more and more outdated history. More and more women are taking on "tough," high-pressure jobs. (The kind of jobs they were thought to be not emotionally strong enough to handle fifty years ago.) On the other hand, more and more men are throwing off the stereotype image and admitting that they are suffering from depression.

POT-SHOTS NO. 4417
Ashleigh Brilliant
ALL I ASK IS THAT YOU CONTINUE INDEFINITELY TO LET ME TAKE ADVANTAGE OF YOUR GOOD NATURE.
©ASHLEIGH BRILLIANT 1988.

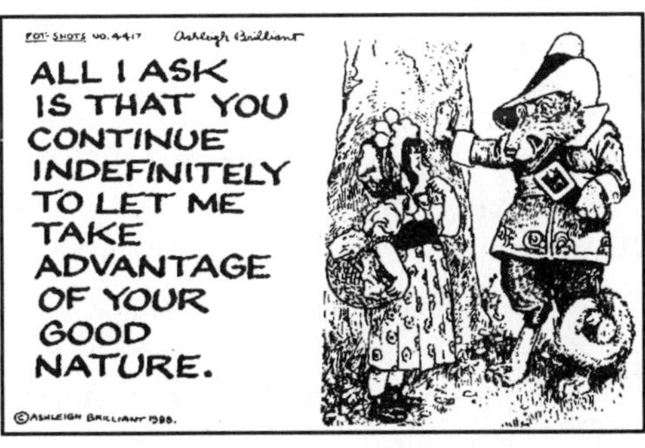

With the explosion of the traditional myth, what is the real truth? Who are more susceptible to depression: men or women?

Statistically, women do, in fact, experience depression roughly twice as often as men. The word "statistically" is emphasized because the traditional myth is not yet completely destroyed and women are still more likely to come forward and admit to feeling depression than men. At the present time, therefore, it is impossible to be absolutely certain.

However, whether or not women are more susceptible to depression than men is hardly significant. What is important is that if you, man or woman, have the misfortune to become acquainted with this illness, the treatment and recovery are at hand. So there is nothing to worry about.

Although the depression (and the suffering) is the same for both men and women, the events which trigger the illness may not be the same on account of their biological differences. During their menstrual cycles women experience hormonal changes which can affect the mood. Some women feel depressed and irritable typically between the time of ovulation and menstruation. This is part of what is called the premenstrual syndrome (PMS) or premenstrual dysphoric disorder (PMDD).

Women (and men) may get depression when they are trying to start a family and find that, despite all efforts, they are unable to have children.

Giving birth and fondling one's new born baby is an event most women look forward to despite the pangs of labor. A common reaction after giving birth is a temporary depression, called postpartum depression or postpartum blues. Surprisingly, some men become depressed after their wives give birth because they feel "left out."

> *The only time a woman really changes a man is when he's a baby.*
> Natalie Wood (1938–1981)

Having an abortion may bring on depression immediately or even years later. Depression sometimes also develops at the approach of the anniversaries of the abortion and the expected birth date of the unborn child.

For most women, these depressions clear up after a few days or weeks. For a minority, usually women who are already prone to depression, the depression may linger and become severe.

When a mother is depressed, she cannot show as much attention to her children as she would like. The atmosphere at home will be subdued and the mother's mood may be infectious. This is especially so if the children are still babies or toddlers and she stays at home all day to look after them. Unfortunately, this may have a negative effect on her children's educational, social and psychological development.

(Of course, this applies equally in reverse when a working mother is out all day and a depressed father stays at home to look after the children.)

Widowhood, divorce and being unmarried also increase the chances of having depression. This applies equally to both men and women. It is a sad fact today that most single parents are women. The situation is particularly distressing when a depressed woman is a single parent, and she and her children have no husband and father respectively to cheer them up and share their life and responsibilities with.

Sexual abuse, molestation and physical abuse, whether as a child or an adult, can also bring on depression. This applies both immediately and later on in life, and to both men and women. Unfortunately, it again is a sad fact of life that far more women are molested than men.

Harassment at work also can bring on depression. Harassment is usually a matter of power, with the victim being a subordinate. At present, women tend to have the junior roles but the situation, fortunately, is changing with more and more women climbing the corporate ladder and taking on high level positions. When that happens, however, men may find themselves the victims. (The next chapter deals with the problem of work induced depression.)

Encouraging is the fact that there is no evidence to show that either pregnancy or menopause are associated with an increased risk of depression. In fact, depressions often diminish during pregnancies.

All these events described in this chapter can happen to any woman. As with any distressing event, the chance of them triggering a full blown depression is much higher when a woman is already disposed to the illness. The important lesson to learn is to recognize when one is depressed, seek treatment and progress towards recovery.

In particular, if you are a woman and know that you are prone to depression, discuss with your doctor whether you should take a small dose of antidepressants or a short course of psychotherapy to get you through situations such as premenstrual syndrome, postpartum depression, alone-all-day-with-baby-and-feeling-miserable, domestic tension, job harassment, etc.

Furthermore, if you are planning on becoming pregnant in the near future and are on an antidepressant, discuss with your doctor whether you should stop taking your medication for a temporary period or switch to another. Fortunately, most antidepressants have no proven adverse effects on pregnancy. Nevertheless, you do not want to take any unnecessary chances and most doctors will recommend you to stop for a while.

CAUSES OF DEPRESSION IN WOMEN

Giving birth is a privilege only women have, an event most look forward to eagerly. Men, for this reason, never experience female depression associated with:

1. Childbirth (postpartum "blues")
2. Premenstrual syndrome (PMS)

The following causes of depression are more common to women than to men:

3. Sexual molestation
4. Physical abuse
5. Single parenthood

I like the dreams of the future better than the history of the past.
Thomas Jefferson (1743–1826)

Chapter 25

Overcoming Work-Related Depression .... and the Problem of Harassment

In the competitive world of work, it is human nature for people to take advantage of others whom they feel are weaker than themselves. Depressed people are especially vulnerable. By nature they are low spirited, tired, feeling worthless, etc. Just the kind of material that unscrupulous and bullying types will choose to pick upon. Worse still, the concentration of depressed people is weaker, they are prone to errors and accidents, self confidence is low, and they tend to give up. Or even feel guilty; because of the illness, not because they really have anything to feel ashamed about. A safe bet for competitive colleagues who want to show they are superior, and domineering managers who want to show they are "in charge."

POT-SHOTS NO. 4591.
CAN A BRUISED EGO
BE CONSIDERED A WORK-RELATED INJURY?
©ASHLEIGH BRILLIANT 1988
Ashleigh Brilliant

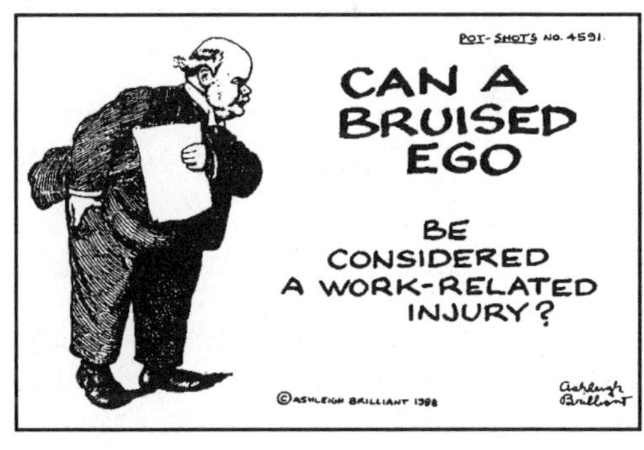

Promotion prospects become dimmer. The depressed person gets stuck in a rut. He (she) comes home exhausted and dejected. The wife (husband) and children sense this and become tense and unhappy as well. Why should this happen?

Bullying at work is like a malignant cancer; it creeps up on one and grows and grows. Like bullying at school, it often takes place where there are no witnesses. Without witnesses it is very difficult to bring concrete proof when making a complaint to one's superiors.

An aggressively competitive colleague may humiliate and undermine a rival by passing on incomplete or partially incorrect details of a project they are supposed to work on together. If found out, he (she) will pass it off as an accidental oversight.

A domineering manager can bully in very subtle ways. For example, he (she) may continually pass over a very able subordinate for promotion. He (she) may take the credit for someone else's work. He (she) may frequently alter goals, knowing that the new objectives cannot be achieved.

Exploitation and verbal abuse are favorite tactics used by the intimidator, humiliating colleagues or subordinates in front of other staff with snide remarks and harsh, repetitive criticism.

The attitude of those at the top of the organization is very important. If they choose not to be firm with an aggressor, then in a way they are condoning the bullying by allowing it to take place. Then they risk losing the respect of valuable employees.

What makes the problem intriguing is the difficulty of distinguishing unfair bullying from reasonable forcefulness to achieve results. Exhortation is desirable and necessary to meet ambitious targets, so long as it is done in a diplomatic manner. Drawing the line between what is and is not acceptable behavior can be tricky. Unfortunately, some company chiefs admire bullies for their "strong personalities."

> *As long as conscience is your friend, never mind about your enemies.*
>
> Anonymous

Work and family life are closely intertwined. When a person is constantly bullied at work, family life is almost certain to become equally stressed.

What can you do if you think you are a victim of bullying? Confrontation is often not safe, even though this approach sounds straightforward and common sense. The person accused may become enraged and even more vindictive than before. The victim (you) will be regarded as "difficult" and branded as a "trouble maker." Challenging the behavior interferes with the bully's complex struggle for power and personal security.

When you the victim are depressed, even mildly, you are even more ill-equipped for confrontation. Therefore, it is most important to take steps to rid yourself of depression. Before taking any action, you must be aware of what is going wrong. Personal survival lies in recognizing what is happening while you are still only slightly affected.

Early warning signs may be detected by asking yourself the following questions:

1. Does the working relationship feel different to how it was previously; e.g., a few months or years ago, or before the new manager took over?
2. Are you persistently being victimized?
3. Although standards have not dropped, is your work constantly being criticized?
4. Are you beginning to wonder whether the mistakes you are supposedly making are really your own fault?

The last may sound surprising or even ridiculous. However, one of the commonest symptoms of depression is taking on guilt, even when not deserved.

If early warning signs are detected, you should ask yourself:

1. Why are things wrong now when everything was all right before?
2. What has changed?
3. Has your organization recently been taken over or reorganized?
4. Has a new manager arrived recently?
5. Is extra pressure being put on your manager?
6. Have you recently moved to a new job?
7. Are your work objectives constantly being altered?
8. Are you being asked to do things outside your job description?
9. Are you being put under more personal scrutiny? Especially intense and critical?
10. Are you being made less involved?

> *Ability will enable a man to get to the top, but character is the only thing that keeps him from falling off.*
>
> Anonymous

It is essential to keep up your spirits at this stage. It may be the intention of the bully (conscious or otherwise) to get rid of you by looking for any reason to accuse you of poor performance which could lead to eventual dismissal. This is what you can do to maintain your self-respect:

1. Stand firm if you come under personal attack. Tell the bully you will not tolerate personal remarks. Do this in private because bullies are reluctant to back down in front of an audience.
2. Keep in mind that the bully is likely to be at his (her) worst when he (she) feels under pressure.
3. Remain confident in your own judgment and ability.
4. Keep calm and say what has to be said quietly and coherently if you clash over work responsibilities.
5. Ask for written clarification ("to serve as a memory guide") if instructions or objectives are unclear. You will have important evidence if things do not improve or goals are changed mid-stream.
6. Try to fathom out the pressures the bully is under, from his (her) own managers. Perhaps he (she) has a difficult domestic life.
7. Review previous annual reports and appraisals to make sure that it is not **your** performance that is slipping. Check with colleagues.
8. Check that you are not being given tasks inconsistent with your job description.
9. Make a detailed record (including dates) of every verbal attack and every new instruction.
10. **Important:** keep copies of all correspondence relating to your job, including memos.

If you decide it is time to fight back:

1. Find out what your company policy or staff handbook says you can do if you feel the time has come to make a complaint. Approach your trade union for advice.
2. Ascertain whether other staff members are being treated similarly to you. The more who experience the same kind of conduct, the less you will be thought of as having a personality clash.
3. Before using official channels, try an informal approach. This is more relaxed and less likely to provoke the bully and backfire on you if it does not work out.

4. Ask a third party (e.g., a trade union, personnel or welfare officer) to inform the bully that people find his (her) behavior aggressive, and the effect it is having.
5. If this produces no results, ask them to put the complaint in writing to the bully, with a copy to his (her) boss if appropriate.
6. Avoid being alone with the bully. Never have meetings together behind closed doors. Always have a witness present.
7. Write a confidential memorandum to senior management above the bully, explaining what is going on and that you trust it will not be allowed to continue.

The clearest indication that something is seriously wrong will be your health. You may already be suffering from depression. If not, bullying is most likely to bring it on. You will feel several or all of the following symptoms:

DEPRESSION AT WORK

Physical symptoms		Emotional symptoms	
1.	nausea	1.	anxiety
2.	palpitations	2.	irritability
3.	indigestion	3.	panic attacks
4.	sweating	4.	crying
5.	disturbed sleep	5.	poor concentration
6.	loss of energy	6.	lack of motivation
7.	severe headaches	7.	little interest or pleasure in various activities
8.	constipation	8.	feeling of isolation
9.	general aches and pains	9.	reduced self esteem
10.	poor appetite	10.	indecisiveness

The stress experienced by those who feel bullied often leads to strained relationships and family tension. It can also cause severe problems related to excessive use of alcohol, drugs, or injuries due to poor concentration, etc.

There is little choice for you if you work in a business or organization run by a bullying manager. There is no one above him (her) to turn to. Handing in your resignation may be the only realistic solution.

What is it that turns a person into a bully? Many psychologists have delved into this question and have come up with various answers:

1. The chain reaction. Brought up in a totalitarian atmosphere, a powerless child is bullied and hit by his (her) father, mother, and older brothers and sisters. It is the beginning of a cycle of violence which starts within the family and moves out. As the child grows up and turns into an adult, he (she) in turn bullies those who are less powerful.

2. Inappropriate anger. This is where a person puts on a show of anger intending to correct an inappropriate course of action and create a beneficial outcome. However, the anger is overdone and the person loses control. This produces an adverse effect.

3. Narcissism. The parent tells the child that he (she) is always wonderful despite any wrongdoing. For example, parents of convicted murderers are often adamant that "their child" is innocent and has committed no crime. The child grows up believing that he (she) can do no wrong and happily persecutes others who do not meet his (her) needs.

> *Any fool can criticize, condemn and complain, and most do.*
> Dale Carnegie in "How to Win Friends and Influence People" (Pocket Books)

4. Sadism. Through constant abuse and bullying, a child's faith in the idea of a benevolent world is eroded by its betrayal. He (she) develops a compulsive attitude characterized by an urge to repeat the experience of being abused. Emerging into adulthood as a tormentor, he (she) feels a constant need to seek situations where he (she) can replicate the experience of tormenting.

5. Insecurity. Many bullies use aggression as a form of self-defence. Basically they feel insecure and afraid of close and intimate relationships. By keeping others at arm's length through aggression, they hope to cover up weak spots and deflect criticism away from themselves.

6. Envy. Where a person, especially a superior, is disconcerted by another person's qualities, abilities and ambitions. He (she) may even feel threatened and deals with it by humiliating and undermining his (her) rival.

7. Seeking love, respect and attention. Some people who are deprived of love in childhood develop a craving for power or a need to be famous. Ambitions are linked to gaining power to compensate for the powerlessness they felt as a child. Ironically, bullying invites rejection, fear and distrust; the opposite of what is intended.

Genuine authority emanates from the respect and commitment a leader evokes. It comes from the trust an employee has in his (her) integrity. Bullying leadership, which controls others by both threatening and carrying out threats, is based on fear. It does not reflect the best management.

Surprisingly, many bullies are vulnerable to bold confrontation, especially those trying to cover up for insecurity. However, bold confrontation requires strength and stamina. For people who are depressed, even mildly depressed, this is cold comfort because they do not have the necessary strength and stamina. By threatening retribution to the victims who stand up, the bullies consolidate their power. They frighten to such an extent that nothing is done and the problem is perpetuated.

On the other hand, many bullies are **not** vulnerable to bold confrontation. They even have a knack of making people who dare stand up to them look silly, as though they are blowing up a problem out of nothing. Then they proceed to put them down. The aggressors make the victims feel as though it is they who have a problem.

POT-SHOTS NO. 4363.
ANYBODY CAN BE WRONG OCCASIONALLY,
Ashleigh Brilliant
BUT ONLY TRULY EXCEPTIONAL PEOPLE CAN MAKE AN ENTIRE CAREER OF IT.
©ASHLEIGH BRILLIANT 1988

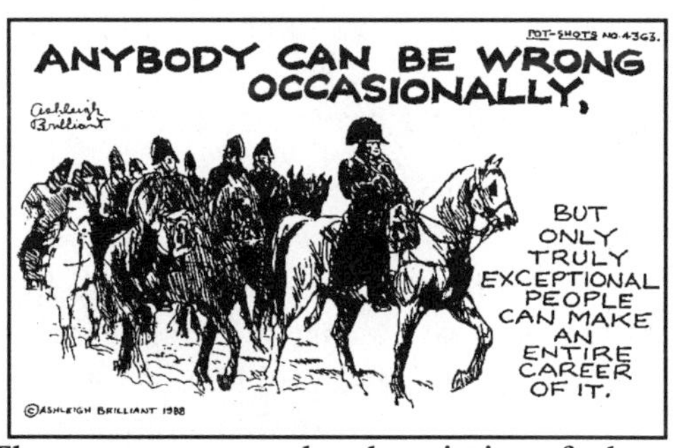

This is why it is important to climb out of the rut by attacking the depression head on. Whether by medication or by therapy, it is essential to have the strength and capability to successfully carry out the decision to do one of the three alternative options: confront the bully, ignore him (her) and weather the storm, or look for another job. And also remain sane!

Attacking the depression should come first, before deciding which option to follow. No important decision should be made while still depressed.

Moreover, bullies do not like picking on people who are high spirited or who look as though they might fight back. On the whole, they would rather choose people whom they perceive as weak and spineless. Other targets are those with good looks, popularity and higher qualifications.

Looking for another job may be a difficult decision. Quitting a well-paid position one may have worked in for many years, giving up career prospects, and leaving friends and colleagues is not something to be done lightly. It has to be very carefully thought over. You may resent the fact that it is **you** who has to leave. Surely, it should be the bully! You may feel as though you are a wimp, losing face, lamely giving up without a fight.

If so, do not! Consider the situation where you choose confrontation. Is it likely to work? Has someone else tried it? What happened? Did matters improve or get worse? Does the bully have friends in high positions and/or a network of sycophants? This lessens your chances of winning. Putting your feelings aside, what are your realistic chances of succeeding? If the answer is "not great," then it is best to put on a brave face and swallow your pride.

Even if you opt for confrontation, there is another important question to ask yourself. Will you be able to survive the pressure? Do you have the strength and stamina? Be honest with yourself. Success at the cost of having a nervous breakdown, continuous ill health, constant stress, and problems with your family (caused by the stress) is not worthwhile. It is a hollow victory. In that case, moving to another job is the most pragmatic and sensible solution.

Getting another job and moving to another organization where you are well treated may be a blessing in disguise. You may actually progress in your career better than you ever thought. Some people find great satisfaction in starting their own business. As the saying goes, every cloud has a silver lining.

HARASSMENT AT WORK: A TEN POINT SURVIVAL PLAN

1. Meet with a welfare officer at work and relate your experiences.
2. Make an appointment with a guidance counselor in your local area.
3. Tell your doctor what is happening to you at work.
4. Make a conscious effort to eat a balanced diet.
5. Take the antidepressants prescribed by your doctor. Discuss with him (her) whether or not to take tranquilizers because they may increase depression and make you less able to maintain a good performance at work.
6. Avoid making any important decisions while depressed.
7. Try to keep your sense of humor.
8. Maintain contact with friends and relatives outside work. You need good listeners. Do not let yourself become isolated.
9. Fight lethargy. However deflated you feel, make time to do things you enjoy outside work hours. Give yourself treats.
10. Attend training courses in assertiveness. They will help you cope.

Remember, no one can make you feel inferior without your consent.
Eleanor Roosevelt (1884–1962)

Chapter 26

Self-help .... 205 Ways to Alleviate Depression

While medication and psychotherapy are helping you to recover from depression, there is nothing like helping yourself at the same time. In fact, the only sure proof of recovery is seeing that you are a full participant in a balanced, active, social and professional life. Medicine and therapy give you the means to do this; the rest is up to you!

©ASHLEIGH BRILLIANT 1983.
POT-SHOTS NO. 2980.
Ashleigh Brilliant
I ORDER YOU TO BE HAPPY!
THE PENALTY FOR DISOBEDIENCE IS: UNHAPPINESS.

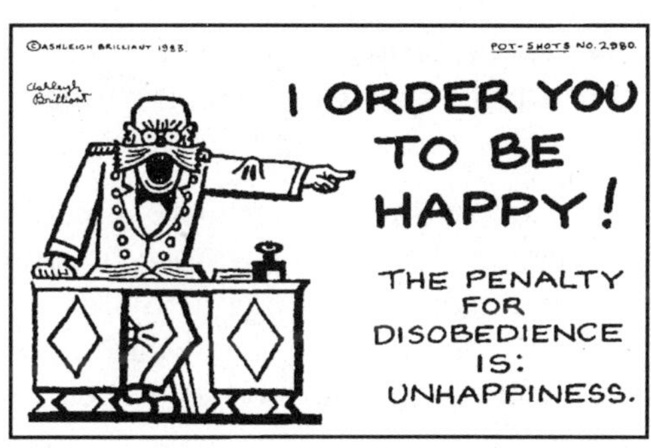

Take up exercise and activities, join self-help groups and clubs, change your lifestyle, let go of circumstances beyond your control, delegate routine, monotonous activities which make you feel depressed, give yourself occasional treats, and get yourself a mentor for advice on domestic and professional affairs. Get immersed gradually and take on more and more until you feel satisfied with the direction your life is taking. It becomes easier and better as you go along.

At the end of this chapter is a potpourri of over two hundred ways in which you can speed yourself to recovery. Pick and choose a mixture which attracts you. As your recovery proceeds, you probably will find yourself becoming interested in more and more of these suggestions. At the same time, you will find yourself picking up and doing things quicker and quicker so you will have more time on your hands to take on extra activities if you so wish.

Certain suggestions are strongly recommended: exercise, a social activity, joining a self-help group and getting yourself a mentor.

Exercise is known to release endorphins in the brain, a natural substance which acts as a mood brightener. Everyone feels more alert after exercise. Social activities are an antidote to depression which dampens one's inclination to mix with other people. This is the way to build up (or even learn) social relationships and develop self-respect.

Research shows that regular workouts relieve depression, raise self-esteem, lessen stress, and sharpen the mind. Even moderate activity helps, say a brisk walk during the lunch break. A swim for thirty to sixty minutes or a jog for three quarters of an hour daily for three months will make a significant difference to the mood and overall sense of well-being.

Long-term exercise may also head off slowed reaction times and loss of short-term memory that often comes with old age. However, no evidence shows that exercise improves mental skills among the young or middle-aged, or that it boosts intelligence at any age.

Sports that are repetitive, predictable, and non-competitive give the best results. Deep rhythmic breathing, such as in swimming and running, induces relaxation. Start with low levels of exercise and gradually build it up without pushing yourself too hard. Keep within reasonable levels; do not set targets so high that you soon give up altogether. Put aside regular times and make exercise a habit.

> *It's not whether you get knocked down, it's whether you get up.*
> Vince Lombardi (1913–1970)

Whenever you have a problem, it is good to talk it over with someone else who has been through something similar. It is comforting to know that you are not alone. In a self-help group people share their experiences and efforts towards recovery with others. Depression is a lonely experience and it is comforting to build up your life with others. Doing things by yourself can be off putting; doing things in a group provides an incentive to succeed. In fact, a self-help group provides a forum for **mutual** help; where everyone helps each other by sharing experiences, information, advice and encouragement.

Self-help groups have four characteristics: their members share common problems and experiences, their members fight for similar goals, they are run for and on behalf of their members, and are not-for-profit. Therefore they are cheap and may serve as a viable alternative to expensive psychotherapy. However, self-help groups should be regarded as a supplement, not a replacement, for professional treatment. This applies especially in the case of severe or long-term depression.

A plethora of self-help groups is available to support both the victims of depression and their families. Some are more widespread than others; others are better organized. Differences may exist between chapters even within the same organization. Therefore, it is impossible to give any recommendations here. The best approach is to attend a few meetings of the various groups in your area and decide for yourself. Consider the following factors: is the group well run, does it offer what you need, is the time and place suitable, and do you feel comfortable with the other people in it?

As explained before, attending the meetings of one of these groups may well be an effective and cheap alternative to psychotherapy. If you do so for this reason, focus on a group which emphasizes positive growth and change. Then see how you feel after about three months. If there has been no worthwhile development in your recovery, try another group until you meet with success.

In the References and Sources (page 243) you will find a list of self-help organizations for depression and related illnesses. Contact those you are interested in who will refer you to your local chapter.

This is a list of the major self-help groups across America but it is by no means exhaustive. Many self-help groups operate only in small, local areas. There may happen to be one in your area which is just right for you. You may be able to find out about them from your local library or your doctor.

> *No man's advice is entirely worthless. Even a watch that won't run is right twice a day.*
>
> Anonymous

Another way to find out the names of all the self-help groups operating in your locality which deal in your area of interest is through a self-help clearinghouse if there happens to be one near to where you live. Unfortunately, they are unevenly distributed and are found in only approximately 20 states. These clearinghouses provide details of both local groups and chapters of national organizations. Some give referrals statewide, others only in the local region. A list is shown in the References and Sources (page 249).

Finally, one cannot overstate the importance of getting yourself a mentor to talk about your domestic and business affairs. It is always a good idea to discuss matters and sound out the opinion of another person you can trust. When you are depressed, you often imagine things are much worse than they really are and see problems out of proportion.

The man who moves a mountain begins by carrying away small stones.

Confucius (551–479 B.C.)

Take your time to choose a mentor (or two) to discuss your problems and affairs. Make sure that the person is in a position to give good advice. For example, a close friend may not be able to give you sound, objective business advice based on experience. Conversely, a business advisor cannot advise you about friends and family whom he does not know. Choose someone who is level-headed and who has been successful in the area where you are seeking advice.

A good source of business advice is a retired business executive. For example, a member of the Service Corps of Retired Executives (SCORE), a part of the federal Small Business Administration's volunteer network. (There is no charge for this service except for small, out-of-pocket expenses.) Many sound businesses fail through poor organization or insufficient planning. A good, competent advisor will warn you of problems and suggest solutions long before they cause problems when it may be too late to put things right. (You cannot afford to let that happen or you will have a real cause for depression!) This kind of advice is extremely valuable and even worth paying for.

Below are 205 ways to alleviate depression and help yourself to a full and speedy recovery:

A. Take up exercise and activities

1. Walking
2. Jogging
3. Running
4. Swimming
5. Ice-skating

6. Mow the lawn
7. Bicycling
8. Gymnastics
9. Exercise machines
10. Aerobics

11. Roller skating
12. Running
13. Basketball
14. Hockey
15. Football

16. Baseball
17. Tennis
18. Ice-hockey
19. Bowling
20. Long walks

©ASHLEIGH BRILLIANT 1983.
POT-SHOTS NO. 3064.
Ashleigh Brilliant
SOME THINGS LEAVE MY LIST AFTER I'VE DONE THEM ~
OTHERS AFTER I'VE ABANDONED HOPE OF DOING THEM.

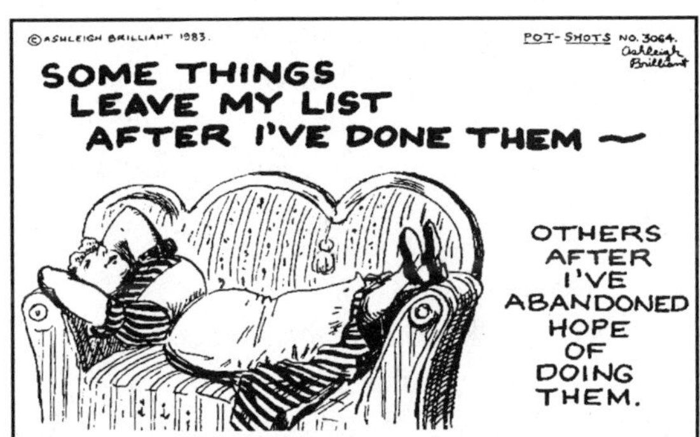

21. Hiking
22. Dancing
23. Yoga, meditation, relaxation techniques
24. Fishing
25. Reading

26. Amateur theater
27. Public speaking
28. Bingo
29. Card games
30. Sex (only if you're up to it. Deep depression may cause sexual dysfunction owing to decreased libido. If so, wait until the depression lifts.)

31. Listening to music at home
32. Going out to concerts
33. Taking up an instrument
34. Singing
35. Performing music in a group

Music washes away from the soul the dust of everyday life.
Berthold Auerbach (1812–1882)

36. Gardening
37. Cookery
38. Restoring historic buildings and sites
39. Assisting in a stately home
40. Volunteering in a museum

41. Guiding people around an historical building
42. Participating in an archaeological dig
43. Cleaning up the environment
44. Long drives with the children or the person you love
45. Cross-country car rallies

46. Needlework
47. Making toys
48. Church/synagogue/mosque: getting involved
49. Helping a charity
50. Politics: campaigning, lobbying, fund raising, etc.

51. Woodwork
52. Metalwork
53. Car repair
54. Boat restoration
55. Building an extension to the home

56. Clay and pottery molding
57. Silkscreen printing
58. Museum visiting
59. Photography
60. Drawing

61. Sketching
62. Painting
63. Sculpturing
64. Modeling
65. Writing books

66. Mailing articles to magazines
67. Authoring a children's book
68. Writing adult fiction stories
69. Composing poetry
70. Writing letters

71. Enrolling in an evening class to develop a skill
72. Practicing a hobby in a group environment
73. Attending a course to learn how to run your own business
74. Canoeing
75. Sailing

76. Kayaking
77. Rowing
78. White water rafting
79. Yachting
80. Motor boating

81. Water-skiing
82. Surfing
83. Looking after a pet
84. Horseback riding
85. Skiing

86. Tobogganning
87. Shopping
88. Going to the theater
89. Watching a ballet
90. Attending an opera

91. An outing to the movies
92. Day trips
93. Weekend jaunts
94. Short breaks with the family
95. Excursions with an organized group

96. Spending time with the children
97. Cleaning your home and furniture
98. Browsing through an outdoor market
99. Watching a sports match on the grounds
100. Watching a video at home

101. Listening to the radio at home
102. Relaxing in front of the television
103. Meditation
104. Yoga

> *To thine own self be true, and it must follow, as the night the day, thou canst not then be false to any man.*
> William Shakespeare (1564–1616)

B. Join a club or self-help group

105. Join a club or committee
106. Become a member of a self-help group

C. Change your lifestyle

107. Take stock of your job
108. Transfer to another department
109. Move to another site in the organization
110. Look for a similar job in another organization

111. Try for that promotion you always wanted
112. Retrain
113. Find a different kind of job
114. Start your own business
115. Work from home

116. Redecorate your home
117. Move the furniture around
118. Swap bedrooms between family members
119. Move to another house or apartment in the locality
120. Move to another house or apartment in a nearby locality

121. Move to another house or apartment far away
122. Move to another state
123. Move to a locality in a better climate
124. Move to a bigger home
125. Move to a smaller home

126. Move to a retirement home
127. Move to a town
128. Move to the countryside
129. Move away from unpleasant neighbors or relatives
130. Move to a district where you can make better friends

131. Move to where there are bigger or better facilities for your children to play in
132. Move somewhere where there are other children for your own to make friends with
133. Relocate where there is a good school your children can attend
134. Look for a new close friend
135. Start dating

136. Get married
137. Separate from your spouse or live-in partner (with whom you are unhappy)
138. Get a divorce (if your marriage is on the rocks)
139. Get a new boyfriend or girlfriend
140. Join a single's group

141. Join an introductions agency or marriage bureau
142. Start dating again
143. Remarry
144. Apply to a school or college
145. Get a degree or professional qualification

146. Change to another school or college (if you are unhappy where you are now)
147. Transfer to a professor you get on better with
148. Transfer to a new course of study
149. Transfer to a different tutoring group
150. Send your child to a different school (a good solution to the problem of bullying classmates, incompetent teachers, or a teaching philosophy you disagree with)

151. Send your child to a larger school (where your child can make more friends and join in more activities)
152. Send your child to a smaller school (where your child can have more individual attention)
153. Change your daily routine
154. Get up earlier in the morning
155. Do some chores before breakfast

156. Change your mealtimes
157. Alter your work schedules
158. Alter your coffee break times
159. Change your recreation times
160. Improve your diet and eating habits

161. Eat more fresh vegetables
162. Consume less fat and more fat-free foods
163. Eat more salads
164. Consume foods with more vitamins and proteins
165. Eat foods with less cholesterol and saturated fats

166. Prepare more cooked meals
167. Eat fewer take-out meals
168. Do your own cooking
169. Prepare gourmet meals
170. Stop consuming TV dinners

171. Get the family to eat meals together
172. Improve your social life
173. Cultivate social friends with new or different interests
174. Expand your circle of friends
175. Go out together for a coffee, tea or ice cream

176. Go out together to sports and recreational events
177. Go out together to the theater or movies
178. Go out together on a fund-raising event
179. Go out together to a restaurant
180. Get yourself a pen pal; write to and meet him (her)

(N.B. Often as one recovers from depression, one becomes more assertive and finds a need for new or different kinds of friends.)

D. Let go of unpleasant activities

181. Minimize monotonous routines in the office
182. Delegate routine, boring tasks to a junior worker
183. Space out monotonous activities throughout the day
184. Hire a cleaning woman at home
185. Buy labor saving devices; e.g., a dishwasher, washing machine and microwave oven

186. Accept changed circumstances
187. Let go of depressing activities
188. Give up commitments or activities you dislike
189. Give up commitments or activities you are not good at
190. Give up commitments or activities you perform less well than your friends or fellow workers

191. Do only those kinds of commitments and activities which you have to do yourself

> *For a man to conquer himself is the first and noblest of all victories.*
>
> Plato (ca. 428–348 B.C.)

E. Give yourself treats

192. Take a vacation
193. Buy yourself some new clothes
194. Buy yourself a new car
195. Purchase a gift for yourself or someone you love.

196. Treat yourself to a luxury
197. Reward yourself when you achieve a goal you set yourself
198. Reward yourself when you manage to complete a chore which is depressing but essential
199. Go out on your birthday
200. Put some spice in your life with a favorite activity

201. Establish highlights to look forward to

F. Get yourself a mentor

202. Get yourself a trusted advisor

203. Cultivate a friend or two with whom you can discuss family and domestic matters, and possibly work problems

204. Find a counselor with whom to discuss serious work problems, domestic affairs and family issues

205. Seek out a business advisor, especially if you are running or plan to start up your own business; e.g., an accountant, lawyer, or experienced businessman

> *Doing your best is more important than being the best.*
>
> Anonymous

PART FOUR:

REFERENCES AND SOURCES

Chapter 27

Drugs That May Cause Depression

Certain medical drugs may produce depressive symptoms. In the following list, only class and generic names are shown.

DRUGS THAT MAY CAUSE DEPRESSION	
Antihypertensives	
Beta-Adrenergic Blocking Agents	Calcium Channel Blockers (cont.)
Acebutolol	Nicardipine
Atenolol	Nifedipine
Betaxolol	Nimodipine
Carteolol	Verapamil
Labetalol	Clonidine
Metoprolol	Doxazosin
Nadolol	Guanfacine
Oxprenolol	Hydralazine
Penbutolol	Hydralazine & Hydrochlorothiazide
Pindolol	Mecamylamine
Propranolol	Methyldopa
Sotalol	Methyldopa & Thiazide Diuretics
Timolol	Metyrosone
Calcium Channel Blockers	Prazosin
Bepridil	Rauwolfia Alkaloids:
Diltiazem	Deserpidine
Felodipine	Rauwolfia Serpentina
Flunarizine	Reserpine
Isradipine	Rauwolfia & Thiazide Diuretics

DRUGS THAT MAY CAUSE DEPRESSION	
Anti-anxiety drugs	
Barbituarates	Benzodiazepines (cont.)
Benzodiazepines	Halazepam
Alprozalam	Ketazolam
Bromazapam	Lorazepam
Chlordiazepoxide	Midazolam
Clonazepam	Nitrazepam
Clorazepate	Oxazepam
Diazepam	Prazepam
Estazolam	Quazepam
Flurazepam	Temazepam
Anti-parkinsonism drugs	
Amantadine	Orphenadrine
Carbidopa & Levodopa	Rimantadine
Levodopa	
Corticosteroids	
Cortisone	
Hormones	
Estrogens (various)	Testosterone & Estradiol
Progestins (various)	
Oral contraceptives	
Desogestrel & Ethinyl Estradiol	Norethindrone & Mestranol
Ethynodiol Diacetate & Ethinyl Estradiol	Norethindrone Acetate & Ethinyl Estradiol
Levonorgestrel & Ethinyl Estradiol	Norgestimate & Ethinyl Estradiol
Norethindrone & Ethinyl Estradiol	Norgestrel & Ethinyl Estradiol

Chapter 28

Mental Health Practitioner Organizations

Besides supplying you with general information, these organizations can give you lists of practitioners and/or let you know whether they are certified to practice.

A list of psychiatrists with qualifications and experience can be obtained from a directory published by the:

American Psychiatric Association (APA)
1400 K Street, NW
Washington
DC 20005 Tel. 202-682-6000

Better still is the annual "Directory of Certified Psychiatrists" published, in collaboration with the American Board of Psychiatry and Neurology, by the:

American Board of Medical Specialties (ABMS)
1007 Church Street, Suite 404
Evanston
IL 60201 Tel. 708-491-9091

A list of psychologists can be obtained from a directory published by the:

American Psychological Association
750 First Street, NE
Washington
DC 20002 Tel. 202-336-5500

An alternative list of state certified or licensed psychologists can be obtained from the:

National Register of Health Service Providers in Psychology
120 G Street, NW, Suite 330
Washington
DC 20005 Tel. 202-783-7663

A list of social workers can be obtained from registers kept by two professional organizations:

National Association of Social Workers, Inc. (NASW)
(Register of Clinical Social Workers)
750 First Street, NE, Suite 700
Washington
DC 20002 Tel. 800-638-8799 or 202-408-8600

American Board of Examiners in Clinical Social Work
3 Mill Road, Suite 306
Wilmington
DE 19806 Tel. 302-739-4522

A list of certified psychiatric nurses can be obtained from:

American Nurses Association
600 Maryland Avenue, SW, Suite 100
Washington
DC 20024 Tel. 202-554-4444

Confirmation of certification of a psychiatric counselor can be obtained from:

National Academy of Certified Clinical Mental Health Counselors
American Mental Health Counselors Association (AMHCA)
5999 Stevenson Avenue
Alexandria
VA 22304 Tel. 703-823-9800 ext. 383

Confirmation of certification of a pastoral counselor can be obtained from:

American Association of Pastoral Counselors
9504A Lee Highway
Fairfax
VA 22031 Tel. 703-385-6967

Other organizations which can assist in choosing a mental health counselor are:

American Family Therapy Association
2020 Pennsylvania Avenue, NW, Suite 273
Washington
DC 20006 Tel. 202-994-2776

American Association of Sex Educators, Counselors and Therapists
435 North Michigan Avenue, Suite 1717
Chicago
IL 60611 Tel. 312-644-0828

National Association of Alcohol and Drug Counselors
1911 North Fort Myer Drive, Suite 900
Arlington
VA 22209 Tel. 703-741-7686

Chapter 29

Useful Information About Drugs for Depression

Notice. While the information on the following pages is true and complete to the best of knowledge, it is intended only as a guide to drugs used for treating medical depression. It is not intended as a replacement for sound medical advice from a doctor. Only a doctor can include the variables of an individual's age, sex, and past medical history needed for wise drug prescription. This chapter does not contain every possible side effect, adverse reaction, or interaction with other drugs or substances. The final decision about a drug's safety or effectiveness must be made by the individual and his (her) doctor. All information, advice, and recommendations in this section are made without guarantees on the part of the author or the publisher, who disclaim all liability in connection with their use.

General guidelines

In order to find out information about a certain antidepressant drug, look up its generic name in the "Drugs: Brand and Generic Names" table on page 165. The tables after that contain the following information:

1. "Drugs: Potential minor side effects" . . . . (pages 166–167)
2. "Drugs: Potential major side effects" . . . . (pages 168–169)
3. "Drugs: Typical overdose symptoms" . . . . (page 170)

When searching these tables, look down the column with the generic name of the drug in which you are interested in order to find out the details specific to it. In addition to doing so, you would find it extremely useful to first read the general guidelines on the next page that apply to all the drugs:

How and when to take: Usually daily, in capsule, liquid, or tablet form.

If you forget a dose: In general, take if you remember within two or three hours. Otherwise, miss out the dose completely.

Time for drugs to take effect: Side effects occur almost immediately. Depression generally begins to lift after approximately two weeks. Full benefit may take more than six weeks to arrive at.

Minor side effects: These usually lessen or disappear as your body adjusts to the medication. Dry mouth can be relieved by chewing gum or sucking on ice cubes. Constipation can be countered with extra fiber in your diet, exercise and more water. Dizziness can be reduced by contracting and relaxing the muscles of your legs shortly before rising, and standing up slowly. Discuss possible side effects with your doctor; also as and when they happen. Note that a person may not get all (or possibly any) of the side effects attributed to a particular drug.

Major side effects: Call your doctor straight away as these may be dangerous. You may need to discontinue the medicine or reduce the dosage.

Discuss with your doctor:

1. If you are taking other medicines; there may be serious interactions
2. Effects of alcohol and tobacco
3. Any foods and drinks to avoid
4. If you have any allergies; or an existing physical or mental illness or condition; or recently had surgery
5. Precautions and side effects if you are over 60 years old
6. If you (or the patient) are an infant or child
7. When you are pregnant, intend to get pregnant, or breast-feed
8. Whether it is safe to drive or operate hazardous machinery
9. What monitoring of the drug is necessary
10. Effects of prolonged use
11. When you discontinue; a gradual reduction may be necessary

DRUGS: BRAND AND GENERIC DRUG NAMES

Common brand name	Generic name
Adapin	Doxepin
Anafranil	Clomipramine
Asendin	Amoxapine
Depakote	Valproate
Depakene	Valproate
Desyrel	Trazodone
Effexor	Venlafaxine
Elavil	Amitriptyline
Endep	Amitriptyline
Lithium (various brands)	Lithium
Ludiomil	Maprotiline
Luvox	Fluvoxamine
Marplan	Isocarboxazid
Nardil	Phenelzine
Norpramin	Desipramine
Pamelor	Nortriptyline
Parnate	Tranylcypromine
Paxil	Paroxetine
Prozac	Fluoxetine
Serzone	Nefazodone
Sinequan	Doxepin
Surmontil	Trimipramine
Tegretol	Carbamazepine
Tofranil	Imipramine
Vivactil	Protriptyline
Wellbutrin	Bupropion
Zoloft	Sertraline

DRUGS: POTENTIAL MINOR SIDE EFFECTS

Symptom / Generic name	Amitriptyline	Amoxapine	Bupropion	Carbamazepine	Clomipramine	Desipramine	Doxepin	Fluoxetine	Fluvoxamine	Imipramine	Isocarboxazid	Lithium	Maprotiline	Nefazodone	Nortriptyline	Paroxetine	Phenelzine	Protriptyline	Sertraline	Tranylcypromin	Trazodone	Trimipramine	Valproate	Venlafaxine
acne				●								●												
agitation						●		●		●						●			●			●		●
anxiety						●			●	●			●		●							●		
appetite loss	●	●	●		●	●	●	●	●	●			●		●	●		●	●			●	●	●
bloating				●								●												
blurred/changed vision						●	●	●		●	●		●	●	●	●	●		●	●	●	●		●
concentration difficulties								●								●			●					●
confusion						●				●			●	●	●							●		
constipation	●	●	●		●	●	●	●		●	●		●	●	●	●	●	●	●	●	●	●	●	●
cramps in stomach	●	●			●	●	●	●		●					●			●				●		
craving of sweet foods											●						●			●				
diarrhea	●	●	●	●	●	●	●	●	●	●	●	●	●	●	●	●	●	●	●	●	●	●	●	●
dizziness	●	●	●		●	●	●	●	●	●	●		●	●	●	●	●	●	●	●	●	●	●	●
drowsiness	●	●		●	●	●	●	●	●	●		●	●	●	●	●		●	●		●	●	●	●
dry mouth	●	●	●		●	●	●	●	●	●	●		●	●	●	●	●	●	●	●	●	●		●
fast heartbeat								●								●			●			●		●
fatigue	●	●	●	●	●	●	●		●	●	●	●	●		●		●	●		●				
flatulence																					●			
flushing								●								●			●					●
frequent urination				●				●	●			●				●			●					●
hair loss																							●	
hand trembling				●								●												
headache			●					●		●						●			●		●		●	●
heartburn	●	●			●	●							●		●			●			●	●		
indigestion							●		●															
insomnia			●			●	●		●	●	●		●		●		●			●		●	●	
irregular heartbeat			●																					
joint/muscle pain																								
light-headedness														●							●			
nausea	●	●	●	●	●	●	●	●	●	●		●	●	●	●	●		●	●		●	●	●	●

DRUGS: POTENTIAL MINOR SIDE EFFECTS																								
Symptom / Generic name	Amitriptyline	Amoxapine	Bupropion	Carbamazepine	Clomipramine	Desipramine	Doxepin	Fluoxetine	Fluvoxamine	Imipramine	Isocarboxazid	Lithium	Maprotiline	Nefazodone	Nortriptyline	Paroxetine	Phenelzine	Protriptyline	Sertraline	Tranylcypromin	Trazodone	Trimipramine	Valproate	Venlafaxine
restlessness	●	●			●	●	●			●	●		●		●		●	●		●		●		
sedation			●						●					●										
sexual disfunction			●					●	●		●					●	●		●	●				●
sleep disorders																					●			
strange dreams																								●
strange tastes	●	●			●	●	●	●	●	●			●		●	●		●	●			●		●
stuffy nose								●								●			●					
sunlight sensitivity	●	●		●	●	●	●			●			●		●			●			●	●		
sweating (excessive)	●	●	●	●	●	●	●	●	●	●	●		●		●	●	●	●	●	●		●		●
thirstiness												●												
tremors									●		●						●			●				
urine turns blue/green	●																							
vomiting	●	●	●	●	●	●	●	●	●	●			●		●			●			●	●	●	
weakness	●	●		●	●	●	●		●	●	●	●	●	●	●		●	●		●		●		
weight gain/loss	●	●			●	●	●	●		●		●	●		●	●		●	●		●	●	●	●

DRUGS: POTENTIAL MAJOR SIDE EFFECTS																								
Symptom / Generic name	Amitriptyline	Amoxapine	Bupropion	Carbamazepine	Clomipramine	Desipramine	Doxepin	Fluoxetine	Fluvoxamine	Imipramine	Isocarboxazid	Lithium	Maprotiline	Nefazodone	Nortriptyline	Paroxetine	Phenelzine	Protriptyline	Sertraline	Tranylcypromin	Trazodone	Trimipramine	Valproate	Venlafaxine
agitation	•	•	•		•		•						•		•			•						
anxiety	•	•			•		•	•								•		•	•					•
balance problems	•	•		•	•	•	•			•			•		•			•				•		
bleeding (unusual)	•	•		•	•	•	•			•					•			•			•	•	•	
blurred vision	•	•	•		•							•						•					•	
breathing difficulties				•				•				•				•			•		•			•
bruising (unusual)	•	•		•	•	•	•			•			•		•			•			•	•	•	
chest pain/tightness	•	•			•	•	•		•	•	•		•	•	•		•	•		•	•	•		
chills				•				•								•			•					•
clumsiness												•												
confusion	•	•			•		•					•						•			•			
convulsions	•	•	•		•	•	•	•	•	•		•	•	•	•	•		•	•			•		•
coordination difficulties	•	•			•	•	•			•			•		•			•			•	•	•	
cramps (stomach)													•										•	
dark urine											•						•			•				
depression				•																			•	
dizziness												•												
edema	•	•			•	•	•			•			•		•			•						
enlarged/painful breasts	•	•			•	•	•			•			•		•			•				•		
eye discomfort				•																				
fainting	•	•		•	•	•	•			•	•	•	•		•		•	•		•		•		
fatigue (extreme)												•												
fever	•	•		•	•	•	•	•		•	•		•		•	•	•	•	•	•		•		•
hair loss	•	•		•	•	•	•			•		•	•		•			•				•		
hallucinations	•	•		•	•	•	•			•	•		•		•		•	•		•	•	•		
headaches	•	•			•	•	•			•	•		•		•		•	•		•		•		
hoarseness												•												
impotence	•	•		•	•	•	•			•			•		•			•				•		
jaundice	•	•		•	•	•	•		•	•	•		•		•		•	•		•		•	•	
joint/muscle pain								•								•			•		•			•
lymph gland swelling								•								•			•					•
menstrual disorders																							•	

DRUGS: POTENTIAL MAJOR SIDE EFFECTS

Symptom / Generic name	Amitriptyline	Amoxapine	Bupropion	Carbamazepine	Clomipramine	Desipramine	Doxepin	Fluoxetine	Fluvoxamine	Imipramine	Isocarboxazid	Lithium	Maprotiline	Nefazodone	Nortriptyline	Paroxetine	Phenelzine	Protriptyline	Sertraline	Tranylcypromin	Trazodone	Trimipramine	Valproate	Venlafaxine
mental disorders																							•	
mood changes	•	•			•	•	•		•	•			•	•	•			•			•	•	•	
mouth sores	•	•		•	•	•	•			•			•		•			•				•		
movement disorders			•																					
nausea											•						•			•				
nervousness	•	•			•	•	•			•			•		•			•				•		
nightmares	•	•		•	•	•	•			•	•				•		•	•		•		•		
nose bleeds						•																		
numbness in fingers/toes	•	•		•	•	•	•			•			•		•			•				•		
palpitations	•	•		•	•	•	•		•	•	•	•	•	•	•		•	•		•	•	•		
prolonged penis erection																					•			
rapid weight gain/loss												•										•		
ringing in ears	•	•		•	•	•	•			•			•		•			•			•	•		
sensitivity to cold												•												
skin dry/rough												•												
skin rash	•	•	•	•	•	•	•	•	•	•	•		•	•	•	•	•	•	•	•	•	•	•	•
sleep disorders	•	•			•	•	•			•			•		•			•				•		
slurred speech											•	•					•			•				
sore throat	•	•		•	•	•	•			•			•		•			•				•		
stiff neck											•						•			•				
swelling of hands/feet				•				•				•			•	•			•					•
swelling of face																							•	
swelling of neck												•												
tingling in fingers/toes				•																	•	•		
tremors	•	•	•		•	•				•		•	•		•		•	•			•	•	•	
twitching				•																				
urinating difficulties	•	•		•		•	•			•	•		•		•		•	•		•	•	•		
urinating pain																					•			
vomiting											•						•			•				
weakness (severe)																					•		•	

DRUGS: TYPICAL OVERDOSE SYMPTOMS

Symptom / Generic name	Amitriptyline	Amoxapine	Bupropion	Carbamazepine	Clomipramine	Desipramine	Doxepin	Fluoxetine	Fluvoxamine	Imipramine	Isocarboxazid	Lithium	Maprotiline	Nefazodone	Nortriptyline	Paroxetine	Phenelzine	Protriptyline	Sertraline	Tranylcypromin	Trazodone	Trimipramine	Valproate	Venlafaxine
agitation			●					●			●						●			●				
breathing difficulties											●						●			●				
cardiac arrhythmias	●	●			●	●	●			●			●		●	●		●			●	●		●
chest pain																					●			
coma	●	●	●	●	●	●	●			●	●	●	●		●		●	●		●	●	●	●	●
confusion			●								●						●			●				
convulsions	●	●	●		●	●	●	●		●	●	●	●	●	●		●	●		●	●	●		●
decreased urination				●																				
dizziness									●		●						●			●				
drowsiness	●	●			●	●	●		●	●			●	●	●	●		●				●		●
enlarged pupils	●	●		●	●	●	●			●					●	●		●				●		●
excitement											●						●			●				
fainting																					●			
fever	●	●			●	●	●			●	●		●		●		●	●		●		●		●
flushed skin				●																				
hallucinations	●	●			●	●	●			●	●		●		●		●	●		●		●		●
heartbeat irregularities											●						●			●				
insomnia											●						●			●				
involuntary movements				●																				
irregular bleeding				●																				
irritability											●						●			●				
low blood pressure				●																				
muscle stiffness													●											
muscle weakness												●												
nausea														●		●								
respiratory failure	●	●			●	●	●			●			●		●			●			●	●		●
restlessness											●						●			●				
stupor				●								●												
sweating (excessive)											●						●			●				
vomiting								●	●			●		●		●								

Chapter 30

List of Eminent Psychiatrists

These psychiatrists, who are widely recognized as being eminent in the field of depression (and similar illnesses), may be able to assist in referring you to a suitable mental health practitioner. Since they are likely to be very busy, it is unlikely that they will be able to treat you personally. It is best that your doctor makes the contact with these doctors or their secretaries. The list is by no means exclusive, and the names of many more well-regarded practitioners may be obtained from reference books such as "The Best Doctors in America" and "The Best Hospitals in America" (available from most public libraries).

N.B. The symbol "**(c)**" appears after the names of psychiatrists who specialize in treating children child and/or adolescents. "**(g)**" appears after those who specialize in treating geriatric patients.

EMINENT PSYCHIATRISTS
Treating depression and similar illnesses

State	Name, Title and Address	
Alabama	Cleveland Kinney, M.D. (g) Department of Psychiatry University of Alabama Hospital 1713 6th Avenue South, C253 Birmingham AL 35233	205-934-6054
Arizona	Alan J. Gelenberg, M.D. Department of Psychiatry University of Arizona School of Medicine University of Arizona Health Sciences Center 1501 North Campbell Avenue Tucson AZ 85724	520-626-6336

EMINENT PSYCHIATRISTS

Treating depression and similar illnesses

State	Name, Title and Address	
California (Los Angeles)	Michael Gitlin, M.D. Department of Psychiatry University of California at Los Angeles Medical Center 300 UCLA Medical Plaza Los Angeles CA 90024	800-825-9989
California (Los Angeles)	Frank Williams, M.D. **(c)** Department of Psychiatry Cedars-Sinai Medical Center 8730 Gracie Allen Drive, Suite 306 Los Angeles CA 90048	213-655-8077
California (Orange)	Justin David Call, M.D. **(c)** Department of Psychiatry University of California Irvine Medical Center 101 The City Drive South Orange CA 92668	714-456-6023
California (Sacramento)	Thomas F. Anders, M.D. **(c)** Department of Psychiatry Davis Medical Center University of California at Sacramento 2315 Stockton Boulevard Sacramento CA 95817	916-734-2784
California (San Diego)	Dilip Jeste, M.D. **(g)** Department of Psychiatry University of California at San Diego 200 West Arbor Drive San Diego CA 92103	619-543-6222

EMINENT PSYCHIATRISTS

Treating depression and similar illnesses

State	Name, Title and Address	
California (San Francisco)	David Ogami, M.D. Department of Psychiatry St. Mary's Hospital and Medical Center 3527 Sacramento Street San Francisco CA 94118	415-775-0781
California (Stanford)	Stewart Agras, M.D. Department of Psychiatry Stanford University School of Medicine 401 Quarry Road Stanford CA 94305	415-723-7107
Colorado	Steven L. Dubovsky, M.D. Department of Psychiatry University of Colarado School of Medicine University of Colarado Health Sciences Center 4200 East Ninth Avenue Denver CO 80262	303-270-8481
Connecticut (New Haven)	Donald J. Cohen, M.D. **(c)** Department of Psychiatry Yale-New Haven Hospital 20 York Street New Haven CT 06504	203-785-5759
Connecticut (West Haven)	Dennis S. Charney, M.D. Department of Psychiatry/116A Veterans Affairs Medical Center 950 Campbell Avenue West Haven CT 06516	203-937-3837

EMINENT PSYCHIATRISTS

Treating depression and similar illnesses

State	Name, Title and Address	
District of Columbia	Jerry M. Wiener, M.D. **(c)** Department of Psychiatry George Washington University Medical Center 2150 Pennsylvania Avenue, NW, Suite 800 Washington DC 20037	202-994-4078
Florida (Miami)	Edwin J. Olsen, M.D. **(g)** Mount Sinai Department of Psychiatry/UM University of Miami School of Medicine 4300 Alton Road/MRI Building, 2nd Floor Miami Beach FL 33140	305-674-2195
Florida (Tampa)	David V. Sheehan, M.D. Department of Psychiatry University of South Florida College of Medicine 3515 East Fletcher Avenue Tampa FL 33613	813-979-3500
Georgia	Charles B. Nemeroff, M.D. Department of Psychiatry Emory University P.O. Box AF Atlanta GA 30322	404-727-8382
Hawaii	John F. McDermott, Jr., M.D. **(c)** Department of Psychiatry Kapiolani Medical Center University of Hawaii 1319 Punahou Street, Room 638 Honolulu HI 96826	808-973-8375

EMINENT PSYCHIATRISTS

Treating depression and similar illnesses

State	Name, Title and Address	
Illinois (Chicago)	Jan Fawcett, M.D. Department of Psychiatry Rush-Presbyterian-St. Luke's Medical Center 1725 West Harrison, Suite 744 Chicago IL 60612	312-942-5372
Illinois (Chicago)	Bennett Leventhal, M.D. (c) Department of Developmental Psychology University of Chicago Medical Center 5841 South Maryland Avenue Chicago IL 60637	312-702-6751
Illinois (Chicago)	Harold Visotsky, M.D. Department of Psychiatry Northwestern Memorial Hospital Superior Street and Fairbanks Court Chicago IL 60611	312-908-8049
Iowa (Iowa City)	Nancy Andreason, M.D., and George Winokur, M.D. Department of Psychiatry University of Iowa Hospital and Clinics 200 Hawkins Drive Iowa City IA 52242	319-356-1348
Kansas	Harriet Lerner, Ph.D., and Flynn O'Malley, Ph.D. (c) Department of Psychiatry The Menninger Foundation 5800 SW Sixth Avenue Topeka KS 66601	800-351-9058

EMINENT PSYCHIATRISTS

Treating depression and similar illnesses

State	Name, Title and Address	
Louisiana	Kenneth M. Sakauye, M.D. **(g)** Department of Psychiatry Touro Infirmary 1401 Fourcher Street New Orleans LA 70115	504-568-2126
Maine	Joseph E. V. Rubin, M.D. **(g)** Department of Psychiatry Maine Medical Center 121 Middle Street Portland ME 04102	207-772-8634
Maryland (Baltimore)	Paul McHugh, M.D. Meyer 4-113, Department of Psychiatry John Hopkins University School of Medicine 600 North Wolfe Street Baltimore MD 21287	410-955-3266
Maryland (Bethesda)	Judith L. Rapaport, M.D. **(c)** Child Psychiatry Branch National Institute of Mental Health 9000 Rockville Pike Bethesda MD 20892	301-496-6080
Maryland (Rockville)	Frederick K. Goodwin, M.D. Mental Health Administration National Institute of Mental Health 5600 Fishers Lane, Room 17-99 Rockville MD 20857	301-443-3673

EMINENT PSYCHIATRISTS

Treating depression and similar illnesses

State	Name, Title and Address	
Massachussetts (Belmont)	Joseph Biederman, M.D. (c) Department of Psychiatry Higginson Building McLean Hospital 115 Mill Street Belmont MA 02178	617-855-3560
Massachussetts (Boston)	Gerald F. Rosenbaum, M.D. Department of Psychiatry Massachussetts General Hospital 15 Parkman Street Boston MA 02114	617-726-3488
Massachusetts (Clinton)	Gary Stuart Moak, M.D. (g) Department of Psychiatry Clinton Hospital 201 Highland Street Clinton MA 01510	508-365-4531
Massachusetts (Springfield)	Benjamin Liptzin, M.D. (g) Department of Psychiatry Baystate Medical Center Springfield MA 01199	413-784-4235
Michigan (Detroit)	Beth Ann Brooks, M.D. (c) Department of Psychiatry Henry Ford Hospital 2799 West Grand Boulevard Detroit MI 48202	313-876-2915
Michigan (Detroit)	Thomas W. Udhe, M.D. Department of Psychiatry Wayne State University Psychiatric Center 2751 East Jefferson Street, Suite 200 Detroit MI 48207	313-993-3416

EMINENT PSYCHIATRISTS

Treating depression and similar illnesses

State	Name, Title and Address	
Minnesota (Minneapolis)	Paula J. Clayton, M.D. Department of Psychiatry University of Minnesota Hospital and Clinic P.O. Box 77 420 Delaware Street, SE Minneapolis MN 55455	612-626-3532
Minnesota (Minneapolis)	Gabe J. Maletta, M.D. **(g)** Department of Psychiatry Minneapolis Veterans Affairs Medical Center One Veterans Drive Minneapolis MN 55417	612-725-3302
Missouri (St. Louis)	George T. Grossberg, M.D. **(g)** Department of Psychiatry St. Louis University Medical Center 1221 South Grand Boulevard St. Louis MO 63104	314-577-8726
Missouri (St. Louis)	Richard E. Mattison, M.D. **(c)** Department of Psychiatry St. Louis Children's Hospital One Children's Plaza St. Louis MO 63110	314-454-2303
Nebraska	Mark Fleisher, M.D., and David Folks, M.D. **(g)** Department of Psychiatry University of Nebraska Medical Center 600 South 42nd Street Omaha NE 68198	402-559-5010

EMINENT PSYCHIATRISTS

Treating depression and similar illnesses

State	Name, Title and Address	
New York (Buffalo)	Marion Zucker Goldstein, M.D. **(g)** Department of Psychiatry State University of New York at Buffalo & Erie County Medical Center 462 Grider Street Buffalo NY 14215	716-898-3630
New York (East Setauket)	Gabrielle A. Carlson, M.D. **(c)** Department of Psychiatry State University of New York at Stony Brook Putnam Hall, Room 168 Stony Brook NY 11794	516-632-8840
New York (New York)	Jack D. Barchas, M.D. Department of Psychiatry New York Hospital-Cornell Medical Center 525 East 68 Street, Room F2321 New York NY 10021	212-746-3770
New York (New York)	Robert N. Butler, M.D. **(g)** Department of Psychiatry Mount Sinai Medical Center One Gustave Levy Place New York NY 10029	212-241-4633
New York (New York)	Magda Campbell, M.D. **(c)** Department of Psychiatry Bellevue Hospital 550 First Avenue New York NY 10016	212-263-6206

EMINENT PSYCHIATRISTS

Treating depression and similar illnesses

State	Name, Title and Address	
New York (New York)	Alexander H. Glassman, M.D., and Frederic M. Quitkin, M.D. New York State Psychiatric Institute Columbia-Presbyterian Medical Center 722 West 168 Street New York NY 10032	212-960-5750 212-960-5784
New York (Rochester)	Eric Douglas Caine, M.D. **(g)** Department of Psychiatry Strong Memorial Hospital University of Rochester Medical Center 300 Crittenden Boulevard Rochester NY 14642	716-275-3574
New York (White Plains)	Cynthia Roberta Pfeffer, M.D. **(c)**, and Barnett Samuel Myers, M.D. **(g)** Department of Psychiatry New York Hospital-Cornell Medical Center 21 Bloomingdale Road White Plains NY 10605	914-997-5721
North Carolina (Chapel Hill)	Arthur J. Prange, Jr., M.D. Department of Psychiatry University of North Carolina School of Medicine University of North Carolina Hospitals 101 Manning Drive, Campus Box 7160 Chapel Hill NC 27599	919-966-1489
North Carolina (Durham)	Bernard J. Carroll, M.D. Department of Psychiatry John Umstead Hospital P.O. Box 3414 Butner NC 27509	919-575-7801

EMINENT PSYCHIATRISTS

Treating depression and similar illnesses

State	Name, Title and Address	
North Carolina (Winston-Salem)	Burton V. Reifler, M.D. (g) Department of Psychiatry North Carolina Baptist Hospital Medical Center Boulevard Winston-Salem NC 27157	910-716-4552
Ohio (Cleveland)	Kathleen Franco, M.D., Michael McKee, M.D., and George Tesar, M.D. Department of Psychiatry Cleveland Clinic Foundation 9500 Euclid Avenue Cleveland OH 44195	216-444-2671 216-444-5816 216-445-6224
Ohio (Columbus)	Henry A. Nasrallah, M.D., and Elizabeth Weller, M.D. (c) Department of Psychiatry Ohio State University Medical Center 410 West 10th Avenue Columbus OH 43210	614-293-8000
Ohio (Dayton)	David G. Bienenfeld, M.D. **(g)**, and William Michael Klykylo, M.D. **(c)** Department of Psychiatry Wright State University School of Medicine Good Samaritan Hospital P.O. Box 927 Dayton OH 45401	513-276-8325
Oklahoma	Betty Pfefferbaum, M.D. (c) Department of Psychiatry Children's Hospital of Oklahoma 940 North East 13 Street Oklahoma City OK 73126	405-271-4274

EMINENT PSYCHIATRISTS

Treating depression and similar illnesses

State	Name, Title and Address	
Ontario, Canada (North York)	George Papatheodorou, M.D. (c), and Duncan Robertson, M.D. (g) Department of Psychiatry Sunnybrook Health Sciences Center 2075 Bayview Avenue North York, Ontario M4N 3M5	416-480-4092 416-480-6802
Ontario, Canada (Toronto)	Harry Moldofsky, M.D., Gary Rodin, M.D., and Brian Shaw, M.D. Department of Psychiatry The Toronto Hospital 585 University Avenue Toronto, Ontario M5G 2C4	416-630-5109 416-603-5766 416-340-3319
Ontario, Canada (Toronto)	Joel Sadavoy, M.D. (g) Department of Psychiatry Mount Sinai Hospital 600 University Avenue, Suite 925 Toronto, Ontario M5G 1X5	416-586-5262
Oregon	Roland Atkinson, M.D. Department of Psychiatry Oregon Health Sciences University Hospital 3181 SW Sam Jackson Park Road Portland OR 97201	503-494-6144
Pennsylvania (Hershey)	Anthony Kales, M.D. Department of Psychiatry Milton S. Hershey Medical Center P.O. Box 850 Hershey PA 17033	717-531-8515

EMINENT PSYCHIATRISTS

Treating depression and similar illnesses

State	Name, Title and Address	
Pennsylvania (Philadelphia)	Salman Akhtar, M.D. Department of Psychiatry Thomas Jefferson University Hospital 1201 Chestnut Street, Suite 1503 Philadelphia PA 19107	215-955-8420
Pennsylvania (Philadelphia)	Barry W. Rovner, M.D. (g) Department of Psychiatry Wills Eye Hospital 900 Walnut Street, 8th floor Philadelphia PA 19107	215-928-3021
Pennsylvania (Philadelphia)	Peter C. Whybrow, M.D. Department of Psychiatry University of Pennsylvania School of Medicine 305 Blockley Hall 418 Service Drive Philadelphia PA 19104	215-662-2818
Pennsylvania (Pittsburgh)	David A. Brent, M.D. (c), and David J. Kupfer, M.D. Department of Psychiatry University of Pittsburgh Medical Center 3811 O'Hara Street Pittsburgh PA 15213	412-624-2353
Quebec, Canada	Herta Guttman, M.D. Department of Psychiatry Royal Victoria Hospital 1025 Pine Avenue West Montreal, Quebec H3A 1A1	514-842-1231 ext. 5314

EMINENT PSYCHIATRISTS

Treating depression and similar illnesses

State	Name, Title and Address	
Rhode Island	Martin B. Keller, M.D. Department of Psychiatry Butler Hospital 345 Blackstone Boulevard, Room 204 Providence RI 02906	401-455-6430
South Carolina	James C. Ballenger, M.D. Department of Psychiatry Medical University of South Carolina 171 Ashley Avenue Charleston SC 29425	803-792-0037
Tennessee (Memphis)	Neil Edwards, M.D. Department of Psychiatry University of Tennessee 66 North Pauline Street, Suite 633 Memphis TN 38105	901-448-6628
Tennessee (Nashville)	Richard A. Margolin, M.D. **(g)**, and Barry Nurcombe, M.D. **(c)** Department of Psychiatry Vanderbilt University Hospital 1161 21st Avenue South Nashville TN 37232	615-322-0325 615-327-7019
Texas (Dallas)	A. John Rush, M.D. Department of Psychiatry University of Texas Western Medical School 5323 Harry Hines Boulevard Dallas TX 75235	214-648-8321

EMINENT PSYCHIATRISTS

Treating depression and similar illnesses

State	Name, Title and Address	
Texas (Galveston)	Robert M. Hirschfeld, M.D. Department of Psychiatry University of Texas Medical Branch Galveston TX 77555	409-772-3901
Texas (Houston)	Charles Milton Gaitz, M.D. **(g)** Department of Psychiatry Bellaire Hospital 6550 Mapleridge Houston TX 77081	713-669-4138
Utah	Paul H. Wender, M.D. Department of Psychiatry University of Utah, 5R154, School of Medicine 50 North Medical Drive Salt Lake City UT 84112	801-581-8075
Virginia	Vamik D. Volkan, M.D. Department of Psychiatry University of Virginia Hospital Jefferson Park Avenue Charlottesville VA 22908	804-924-9001
Washington (Seattle)	David L. Dunner, M.D. Department of Psychiatry University of Washington Medical Center P.O. Box 354794 Seattle WA 98195	206-543-6768
Washington (Seattle)	Richard A. Gode, M.D. **(c)** Department of Psychiatry Virginia Mason Medical Center P.O. Box 900 Seattle WA 98111	206-821-8004 206-625-7404

EMINENT PSYCHIATRISTS

Treating depression and similar illnesses

State	Name, Title and Address	
Washington (Seattle)	Michael J. Norden, M.D. Department of Psychiatry University of Washington Medical Center ℅ 10740 Meridian Avenue North, Suite 101 Seattle WA 98133	206-361-7696
Washington (Tacoma)	Hugo Van Dooren, M.D. Department of Psychiatry Puget Sound Hospital 215 South 36 Street Tacoma WA 98408	206-474-0561 206-627-8448
West Virginia (Morgantown)	Dianne W. Trumbull, M.D. **(c)** Department of Psychiatry West Virginia University School of Medicine Chestnut Ridge Hospital 930 Chestnut Ridge Road Morgantown WV 26505	304-293-2411
West Virginia (Parkersburg)	John Frederic Kelley, M.D. **(c)** Department of Psychiatry Center for Behavioral Medicine ℅ 600 Eighteenth Street, Suite 611 Parkersburg WV 26101	304-424-4670
Wisconsin	Kenneth Johnson, M.D. Department of Psychiatry St. Mary's Hill Hospital 2350 North Lake Drive Milwaukee WI 53211	414-291-1661

Chapter 31

Mental Health Treatment Centers: Directories of Facilities

Besides publishing directories listing hospitals and care centers, the organizations below can supply general information.

1. "The American Hospital Association Guide to the Health Care Field" published by:

American Hospital Association
1 North Franklin Street
Chicago
IL 60606 Tel. 800-242-2626 or 312-422-3000

2. "Mental Health Directory" published by:

U.S. Department of Health and Human Services
(Institute of Mental Health)

and available from:

Superintendent of Documents
Government Printing Office
P.O. Box 371954
PA 15250 Tel. 202-512-1800

Chapter 32

1996 Clinical Studies Related to Depression

1996 CLINICAL STUDIES RELATED TO DEPRESSION Funded and Conducted by the National Institute of Mental Health at Bethesda, MD (near Washington, D.C.)	
Clinical Director	David R. Rubinow, M.D.
Contact Section & Telephone Number	Ms. Nazli Haq, M.A. Office of the Clinical Director National Institute of Mental Health Building 10, Room 3N238 10 CENTER DR MSC 1276 Bethesda MD 20892-1276 Tel. 301-402-0826
1996 Studies	1. Unipolar disorder (depression) 2. Bipolar disorder (manic depression) 3. Seasonal affective disorder (SAD) 4. Obsessive-compulsive and anxiety disorders 5. Borderline personality disorder 6. Disorders of attention and cognition 7. Rapid cycling mood disorders 8. Childhood mental illness 9. Developmental psychology 10. Anxiety disorders 11. Depression and pregnancy 12. Menstrual and menopausal mood and behavioral disorders 13. Alzheimer's disease 14. Genetic studies 15. Alternative medicine and behavioral disorders

OTHER NATIONAL INSTITUTES OF HEALTH

Which may be conducting studies relevant to depression

Name and Clinical Director	Contact Section & Telephone
National Institute on Aging Deputy Director: Mark B Schapiro, M.D.	Patient referrals: Ms. Carol J. Fuchs-Kinslow, MSSW Social Worker Tel. 301-496-4754 Public inquiries: Tel. 301-496-1752
National Institute on Alcohol Abuse and Alcoholism Director: Enoch Gordis, M.D.	Patient referrals: Ms. Irene Culver Tel. 301-496-1993 Public inquiries: Tel. 301-443-3860
National Institute on Child Health and Human Develop-ment Director: Fernando Cassorla, M.D.	Patient referrals: Stephen J. Suomi, Ph.D. Chief of Comparative Ethology (Developmental Psychology Program) Tel. 301-496-9550 General and public inquiries: Tel. 301-496-5133
National Institute on Drug Abuse Director: Alan I. Leshner, Ph.D.	Patient referrals: Recruitment Unit Tel. 410-550-1502 Public inquiries: National Clearinghouse for Alcohol and Drug Information Tel. 800-729-6686

Chapter 33

Institutions Funded by NIH on Projects Related to Depression (1996)

Thousands of doctors throughout the United States receive research money and may be able to treat your illness free of charge. The National Institutes of Health (Division of Research Grants) can help you locate an institution which receives money to conduct research and where you may be able to be treated free of charge. Contact:

The Division of Research Grants
National Institutes of Health
6701 Rockledge Drive, MSC 7762, Suite 3032
Bethesda
MD 20892 Tel. 301-435-0714

Ask for a search of the CRISP (Computer Retrieval for Information on Scientific Projects) database. This search, conducted free of charge, will provide you with the study title, researcher, organization, grant amount, and detailed description of the research project.

NIH FUNDED INSTITUTIONS 1996 On Projects Related to Depression		
State	**City**	**Institution**
Alabama	Birmingham	University of Alabama at Birmingham
Alaska	—	—
Arizona	Tucson	University of Arizona
Arkansas	Little Rock	University of Arkansas
California	Berkeley	University of California at Berkeley
	Irvine	University of California at Irvine
	Los Angeles	University of California at Los Angeles
		University of Southern California

NIH FUNDED INSTITUTIONS 1996 On Projects Related to Depression		
State	**City**	**Institution**
California (cont.)	Oakland	Children's Hospital Medical Center
		Kaiser Foundation Research Institute
	San Diego	University of California at San Diego
	San Francisco	University of California at San Francisco
	Santa Monica	Rand Corporation
	Stanford	Stanford University
	Torrance	Research and Education Institute, Inc.
Colorado	Boulder	University of Colarado at Boulder
	Denver	University of Colarado Health Sciences Center
		University of Denver
Connecticut	New Haven	Yale University
Delaware	—	—
District of Columbia	Washington	George Washington University
		Georgetown University
		Howard University
Florida	Gainesville	University of Florida
	Miami	University of Miami
	Tampa	University of South Florida
Georgia	Atlanta	Emory University
	Augusta	Medical College of Georgia
Hawaii	—	—
Idaho	—	—
Illinois	Champaign	University of Illinois at Urbana-Champaign
	Chicago	Loyola University of Chicago
		Rush-Presbyterian-St. Lukes Medical Center
		University of Illinois at Chicago

NIH FUNDED INSTITUTIONS 1996
On Projects Related to Depression

State	City	Institution
Illinois (cont.)	Evanston	Northwestern University
	Maywood	Loyola University Medical Center
Indiana	Indianapolis	Indiana University - Purdue University at Indiananapolis
		Larue D. Carter Memorial Hospital
	Notre Dame	University of Notre Dame
Iowa	Ames	Iowa State University of Science and Technology
	Iowa City	University of Iowa
Kansas	—	—
Kentucky	—	—
Louisiana	Shreveport	Louisiana State University Medical Center
Maine	—	—
Maryland	Baltimore	John Hopkins University
		Individual Monitoring Systems, Inc.
		Kennedy Krieger Research Institute, Inc.
		University of Maryland at Baltimore
	Greenbelt	American Association for Geriatric Psychiatry
Massachusetts	Belmont	McLean Hospital
	Boston	Brigham and Women's Hospital
		Children's Hospital (Boston)
		Harvard University
		Judge Baker Children's Center
		Massachusetts General Hospital
		New England Deaconess Hospital
		University of Massachussetts
	Newton	Boston College

NIH FUNDED INSTITUTIONS 1996 On Projects Related to Depression		
State	**City**	**Institution**
Michigan	Ann Arbor	University of Michigan at Ann Arbor
	East Lansing	Michigan State University
Minnesota	Minneapolis	University of Minnesota at the Twin Cities
Mississippi	Jackson	University of Mississippi Medical Center
Missouri	St. Louis	Washington University
Montana	—	—
Nebraska	Lincoln	University of Nebraska at Lincoln
Nevada	—	—
New Hampshire	—	—
New Jersey	Belle Mead	Carrier Foundation (Belle Mead, New Jersey)
	Gibbsboro	Dolphin, Inc.
	New Brunswick	Rutgers State University at New Brunswick
	Newark	University of Medicine and Dentistry of New Jersey
New Mexico	Albuquerque	University of New Mexico at Alberquerque
New York	Buffalo	State University of New York at Buffalo
	Elmhurst	Mount Sinai School of Medicine
	Mineola	Winthrop University Hospital
	New Hyde Park	Long Island Jewish Medical Center
	New York City	Columbia University
		Cornell University Medical Center
		Health Sciences Center at Brooklyn
		Mount Sinai School of Medicine
		New York State Psychiatric Institute
		Yeshiva University

NIH FUNDED INSTITUTIONS 1996 On Projects Related to Depression		
State	**City**	**Institution**
New York (cont.)	Rochester	University of Rochester
	Stony Brook	State University of New York at Stony Brook
North Carolina	Chapel Hill	University of North Carolina at Chapel Hill
	Durham	Duke University
	Greensboro	Bennett College
	Winston-Salem	Wake Forest University
North Dakota	—	—
Ohio	Cleveland	Case Western Reserve University
	Columbus	Ohio State University
	Dayton	Wright State University
Oklahoma	—	—
Ontario, Canada	London	University of Western Ontario
Oregon	Eugene	Oregon Research Institute
		University of Oregon
	Portland	Kaiser Foundation Research Institute
		Oregon Health Sciences University
Pennsylvania	Philadelphia	Hahnemann University
		Medical College of Pennsylvania
		Philadelphia Geriatric Center-Friedman Hospital
		Temple University
		Thomas Jefferson University
		University of Pennsylvania
	Pittsburgh	Allegheny General Hospital (Pittsburgh)
		Clinical Tools, Inc.
		MPC Corporation
		University of Pittsburgh at Pittsburgh

NIH FUNDED INSTITUTIONS 1996 On Projects Related to Depression		
State	**City**	**Institution**
Puerto Rico	San Juan	University of Puerto Rico, Rio Piedras
Rhode Island	East Providence	Emma Pendleton Bradley Hospital
	Providence	Brown University
		Butler Hospital
		Rhode Island Hospital
South Carolina	Charleston	Medical University of South Carolina
	Columbia	University of South Carolina at Columbia
South Dakota	—	—
Tennessee	Nashville	Vanderbilt University
Texas	Dallas	University of Texas South West Medical Center at Dallas
	Houston	University of Texas South West Medical Center at Houston
	Lubock	Texas Technical University
	San Antonio	University of Texas Health Sciences Center at San Antonio
Utah	Salt Lake City	Brigham Young University
		University of Utah
Vermont	Winooski	Bio-Tek Instruments, Inc.
Virginia	Charlottesville	University of Virginia at Charlottesville
	Richmond	Virginia Commonwealth University
Washington	Cheney	Eastern Washington University
	Pullman	Washington State University
	Seattle	Center for Health Studies
		University of Washington
West Virginia	—	—
Wisconsin	Madison	University of Wisconsin at Madison
Wyoming	—	—

Chapter 34

Free Health Care at Your Hospital

For information on the Hill-Burton program, including eligibility requirements, facilities required to provide assistance in your area, and complaint procedures, contact:

Bureau of Health Resources Development
Health Resources and Services Administration
Department of Health and Human Services
5600 Fishers Lane, Room 7-31
Rockville
MD 20857
Tel. 800-638-0742 outside MD
Tel. 800-492-0359 inside MD

Chapter 35

State Departments of Public Health

For local free health clinics contact your local State Department of Public Health.

STATE DEPARTMENTS OF PUBLIC HEALTH		
Alabama	Department of Public Health 434 Monroe Street Montgomery AL 36130	334-613-5200
Alaska	Department of Health and Social Services P.O. Box 110650 Juneau AK 99811	907-465-3090
Arizona	Department of Health Services 2122 East Highland Avenue, Suite 100 Phoenix AZ 85016	602-381-8990
Arkansas	Department of Health 3915 West 8 Street Little Rock AR 72204	501-280-3100
California	Department of Health Services 714 P Street Sacramento CA 95814	916-445-4171
Colorado	Department of Health (Family Health Line) 4300 Cherry Creek Drive South Denver CO 80222	800-688-7777 303-692-2229
Connecticut	Department of Health Services 150 Washington Street Hartford CT 06106	203-566-2038

STATE DEPARTMENTS OF PUBLIC HEALTH		
Delaware	Division of Public Health P.O. Box 637 Dover DE 19903	302-739-4701
District of Columbia	Commission of Public Health 1660 L Street NW Washington DC 20036	202-727-1765
Florida	Health and Rehabilitative Services Department 1317 Winewood Boulevard, Building 1, Room 115 Tallahassee FL 32399	904-487-2705
Georgia	Public Health Division Department of Human Resources 2 Peachtree Street, NW Atlanta GA 30303	404-657-2700
Hawaii	Department of Health P.O. Box 3378 Honolulu HI 96801	808-548-6505
Idaho	Department of Health and Welfare P.O. Box 83720 Boise ID 83720	208-334-5500
Illinois	Department of Public Health 535 West Jefferson Street Springfield IL 62761	217-524-5989
Indiana	State Board of Health 1330 West Michigan Street Indianapolis IN 46206	317-232-1000
Iowa	Department of Public Health Lucas State Office Building 321 East 12 Street Des Moines IA 50319	515-281-5605

STATE DEPARTMENTS OF PUBLIC HEALTH

Kansas	Department of Health and Environment Landon Office Building 900 Southwest Jackson Street Topeka KS 66612	913-296-1343
Kentucky	Department of Health Services 275 East Main Street Frankfort KY 40621	502-564-3970
Louisiana	Office of Public Health 325 Loyola Avenue New Orleans LA 70112	504-568-5050
Maine	Department of Human Services 151 Capitol Street State House Station #11 Augusta ME 04333	207-287-3201
Maryland	Department of Health and Mental Hygiene 201 West Preston Street Baltimore MD 21201	410-225-6500
Massachusetts	Department of Public Health 250 Washington Street Boston MA 02108	617-624-5200
Michigan	Department of Public Health 3423 Martin Luther King Junior Boulevard Lansing MI 48909	517-335-8024
Minnesota	Department of Health 717 Delaware Street, SE Minneapolis MN 55440	612-623-5000
Mississippi	Department of Health 2423 North State Street Jackson MS 39215	601-960-7635

STATE DEPARTMENTS OF PUBLIC HEALTH		
Missouri	Department of Health P.O. Box 570 Jefferson City MO 65102	314-751-6001
Montana	Health Policy and Services Division Department of Public Health and Human Services Cogswell Building Helena MT 59620	406-444-4473
Nebraska	Department of Health 301 Centennial Mall South P.O. Box 95007 Lincoln NE 68509	402-471-2133
Nevada	Department of Human Resources, Health Division 505 East King Street, Room 201 Carson City NV 89710	702-687-4740
New Hampshire	Department of Health and Welfare 6 Hazen Drive Concord NH 03301	603-271-4501
New Jersey	Department of Health CN 360 Trenton NJ 08625	609-292-7837
New Mexico	Department of Health 1190 St. Francis Drive Sante Fe NM 87502	505-827-2613
New York	Department of Health Empire State Plaza Albany NY 12237	518-474-2011
North Carolina	Environment, Health and Natural Resources 512 North Salisbury Street Raleigh NC 27604	919-733-4984

STATE DEPARTMENTS OF PUBLIC HEALTH		
North Dakota	Department of Health 600 East Boulevard Bismarck ND 58505	701-328-2372
Ohio	Department of Health 246 North High Street P.O. Box 118 Columbus OH 43266	614-466-2253
Oklahoma	Department of Health 1000 NE 10 Street Oklahoma City OK 73117	405-271-4200
Oregon	Department of Human Resources, Health Division 800 Northeast Oregon Street Portland Oregon OR 97232	503-731-4000
Pennsylvania	Department of Health 802 Health and Welfare Building Harrisburg PA 17120	717-787-6436
Rhode Island	Department of Health 3 Capitol Hill Providence RI 02908	401-277-2577
South Carolina	Department of Health and Environment Control 2600 Bull Street Columbia SC 29201	803-734-4880
South Dakota	Department of Health Anderson Building 445 East Capitol Street Pierre SD 57501	605-773-3361
Tennessee	Department of Health Cordell Hull Building, 3rd Floor 4265 Avenue North Nashville TN 37247	615-741-3111

STATE DEPARTMENTS OF PUBLIC HEALTH

Texas	Department of Health 1100 West 49 Street Austin TX 78756	512-458-7111
Utah	Department of Health 288 North 1460 West Street Salt Lake City UT 84116	801-538-6111
Vermont	Department of Health 108 Cherry Street P.O. Box 70 Burlington VT 05402	802-863-7280
Virginia	Department of Health 1500 East Main Street, Room 214 Richmond VA 23219	804-786-3561
Washington	Department of Health 1112 Southeast Quince Street P.O. Box 47890 Olympia WA 98504	360-753-5871
West Virginia	Health and Human Resources Department Capitol Complex, Building 3, Room 206 Charleston WV 25305	304-558-0684
Wisconsin	Health and Social Services Department 1 West Wilson Street Madison WI 53703	608-266-1511
Wyoming	Department of Health Hathaway Building Cheyenne WY 82002	307-777-7656

Chapter 36

Medicaid and Medicare

For details of federal and state medical programs, contact:

1. Medicare Hotline
   Healthcare Financing Administration
   7500 Security Boulevard
   Baltimore
   MD 21244 Tel. 800-638-6833

2. Medicaid Hotline
   Healthcare Financing Administration
   7500 Security Boulevard
   Baltimore
   MD 21244 Tel. 410-786-7144

These hotlines will give out information and booklets about Medicare and Medicaid respectively. Another source of information concerning free care for children, adolescents and pregnant mothers is the Maternal and Child Health Care Division of your state Department of Public Health (see next chapter).

Chapter 37

State Departments of Public Health: Maternal and Child Health Care Contacts

To find out whether free health care is available for children, adolescents and pregnant mothers locally, contact the Maternal and Child Health Care Division of your state Department of Health.

STATE DEPARTMENTS OF PUBLIC HEALTH Maternal and Child Health Care Contacts		
Alabama	Maternal and Infant Care 434 Monroe Street Montgomery AL 36130	334-242-5766
	Information Referral:	334-242-5661
Alaska	Division of Public Assistance Department of Health and Social Services P.O. Box 110650 Juneau AK 99811	907-465-3347
Arizona	Community Information Referral 1515 East Osbourne (The Annex) Phoenix AZ 85014	602-263-8856
	Information Referral:	800-352-3792
Arkansas	Section of Maternal and Child Health Department of Health 4815 West Markham Street Little Rock AR 72205	501-661-2251
	Information Referral:	800-336-4797

STATE DEPARTMENTS OF PUBLIC HEALTH

Maternal and Child Health Care Contacts

State	Contact	Phone
California	Maternal and Child Health Department of Health Services 714 P Street, Room 750 Sacramento CA 95814	916-657-1347
	Information Referral:	800-222-9999
Colorado	Family Healthline Department of Health 4300 Cherry Creek Drive South Denver CO 80222	303-692-2229
	Information Referral:	800-688-7777
Connecticut	Association for Human Services 880 Asylum Avenue Hartford CT 06105	203-522-7762
Delaware	Division of Public Health 805 River Road Dover DE 19901	302-739-4726
	Information Referral:	800-451-4357
District of Columbia	Office of Maternal and Child Health Commission of Public Health 1660 L Street NW, Suite 907 Washington DC 20036	202-727-0393
	Information Referral:	800-666-2229
Florida	Maternal and Child Health Health and Rehabilitative Services Department 1317 Winewood Boulevard Tallahassee FL 32399	904-487-2705
	Information Referral:	800-451-2229

STATE DEPARTMENTS OF PUBLIC HEALTH

Maternal and Child Health Care Contacts

Georgia	Family Health Services Section Public Health Division Department of Human Resources 2 Peachtree Street, 8th Floor Atlanta GA 30303	404-657-2850
	Information Referral:	800-228-9173
Hawaii	Maternal and Child Health Branch Department of Health 741-A Sunset Avenue Honolulu HI 96816	808-733-9033
	Information Referral:	808-275-2000
Idaho	Idaho WIC Program Bureau of Clinical and Preventive Services Department of Health and Welfare P.O. Box 83720 Boise ID 83720	208-334-5948
	Information Referral:	800-926-2588
Illinois	Maternal and Child Health Department of Public Health 535 West Jefferson Street Springfield IL 62761	217-782-4977
Indiana	Division of Maternal and Child Health State Board of Health 3838 North Rural Street Indianapolis IN 46205	317-541-2313
	Information Referral:	800-433-0746
Iowa	Maternal and Child Health Division Department of Public Health Lucas State Office Building Des Moines IA 50319	515-281-3126
	Information Referral:	800-369-2229

STATE DEPARTMENTS OF PUBLIC HEALTH

Maternal and Child Health Care Contacts

State	Contact	Phone
Kansas	IM-EPS Commission Docking State Office Building 915 Southwest Harrison Street, Room 651W Topeka KS 66612	913-296-3349
	Information Referral:	800-658-4690
Kentucky	Division of Maternal and Child Health Department of Health Services 275 East Main Street Frankfort KY 40621	502-564-3970
	Information Referral:	800-372-2973
Louisiana	Office of Public Health 325 Loyola Avenue New Orleans LA 70112	504-568-5051
	Information Referral:	800-256-4609
Maine	Community and Family Health Department of Human Services 151 Capitol Street, Station #11 Augusta ME 04333	207-287-3311
	Information Referral:	800-698-3624
Maryland	Department of Health and Mental Hygiene 201 West Preston Street, Room 135 Baltimore MD 21201	401-225-6538
	Information Referral:	800-456-8900
Massachusetts	Bureau of Family and Community Health Department of Public Health 250 Washington Street Boston MA 02108	617-624-5070

STATE DEPARTMENTS OF PUBLIC HEALTH

Maternal and Child Health Care Contacts

State	Contact	Phone
Massachusetts (cont.)	Information Referral:	
	Boston Region	800-531-2229
	Central Region	800-227-7748
	Northeast Region	800-992-1895
	Southeast Region	800-642-4250
	West Region	800-992-6111
Michigan	Bureau of Community Health Services Department of Public Health 3423 Martin Luther King Junior Boulevard P.O. Box 30195 Lansing MI 48909	517-335-8945
	Information Referral:	800-262-4784
Minnesota	Department of Human Services 444 Lafayette Road St. Paul MN 55155	612-296-6117
	Information Referral:	
	Maternal & Child Health:	800-657-3672
	Health & Human Services:	800-652-9747
Mississippi	Department of Health 2423 North State Street Jackson MS 39215	601-960-7484
	Information Referral:	800-222-7622
Missouri	Division of Child and Family Health Care Department of Health 1738 East Elm Street Jefferson City MO 65102	314-751-6001
	Information Referral:	800-835-5465
Montana	Health Services Division Health and Environment Sciences Cogswell Building Helena MT 59620	406-444-4740
	Information Referral:	800-762-9891

STATE DEPARTMENTS OF PUBLIC HEALTH

Maternal and Child Health Care Contacts

State	Contact	Phone
Nebraska	Maternal and Child Health Department of Health 301 Centennial Mall South P.O. Box 95007 Lincoln NE 68509	402-471-2907
	Information Referral:	800-862-1889
Nevada	Family Health Services Nevada Health Division Department of Human Resources 505 East King Street, Suite 200 Carson City NV 89710	702-687-4897
	Information Referral:	800-992-0900 ext. 4897
New Hampshire	Helpline 2 Industrial Park Drive Concord NH 03301	603-225-9000
	Information Referral:	800-852-3388
New Jersey	Maternal and Child Health Department of Health 50 East State Street, 6th Floor, CN364 Trenton NJ 08625	609-292-5616
	Information Referral:	800-328-3838
New Mexico	Department of Health 1190 St. Francis Drive Sante Fe NM 87502	505-827-2613
	Information Referral:	800-552-8195
New York	"Growing Up Healthy" Department of Health Perinatal Health Unit, Room 780 Empire State Plaza Albany NY 12237	518-474-1964
	Information Referral:	800-522-5006

STATE DEPARTMENTS OF PUBLIC HEALTH

Maternal and Child Health Care Contacts

State	Contact	Phone
North Carolina	Care Line Department of Human Resources 325 North Salisbury Street Raleigh NC 27603	919-733-4261
	Information Referral:	800-662-7030
North Dakota	Division of Maternal and Child Health Department of Health State Capitol 600 East Boulevard Bismarck ND 58505	701-328-2493
	Information Referral:	800-472-2286
	Children with Special Health Care Needs Department of Human Services State Capitol 600 East Boulevard Bismarck ND 58505	701-328-2436
	Information Referral:	800-472-2622 ext. 2436
Ohio	Bureau of Maternal and Child Health Department of Health 246 North High Street P.O. Box 118 Columbus OH 43266	614-466-5332
	Information Referral:	800-6274-2229
Oklahoma	"Health Line" Department of Health 1000 Northeast 10 Street Oklahoma City OK 73117	405-271-4200
Oregon	Department of Human Resources, Health Division 800 Northeast Oregon Street Portland Oregon OR 97232	503-731-4000

STATE DEPARTMENTS OF PUBLIC HEALTH

Maternal and Child Health Care Contacts

Oregon (cont.)	Information Referral: Safe Net Multnamah County 426 SW Stark Portland OR 97204	800-SAFE-NET
Pennsylvania	"Health Hotline" Department of Health Division of Health Promotion P.O. Box 90, Room 1003 Health and Welfare Building Harrisburg PA 17120	717-787-5900
	Information Referral:	800-692-7254
Rhode Island	(For pregnant mothers and infants only:) "Right Start" Department of Health 3 Capitol Hill, Room 302 Providence RI 02908	401-277-2577
	Information Referral:	800-346-1004
South Carolina	(For pregnant mothers and infants only:) Department of Health First Nine Care Line—MH Robert Mills Complex Columbia SC 29211	803-734-3350
	Information Referral:	800-868-0404
South Dakota	Maternal and Child Health Care Department of Health Anderson Building 445 East Capitol Street Pierre SD 57501	605-773-3737
	Information Referral:	800-658-3080

STATE DEPARTMENTS OF PUBLIC HEALTH

Maternal and Child Health Care Contacts

State	Contact	Phone
Tennessee	Maternal and Child Health Section Department of Health and Environment Tennessee Tower, 10th Floor 312 8 Avenue North Nashville TN 37247	615-741-7353
	Information Referral:	800-428-2229
Texas	Maternal and Child Health Department of Health 1100 West 49 Street Austin TX 78756	512-458-7700
	Information Referral:	800-422-2956
Utah	Maternal and Infant Health Department of Health 288 North 1460 West Street Salt Lake City UT 84116	801-538-6161
	Information Referral:	800-822-2229
Vermont	Department of Health 108 Cherry Street P.O. Box 70 Burlington VT 05402	802-863-7280
	Information Referral:	800-649-4357
Virginia	Department of Health 1500 East Main Street, Room 137 Richmond VA 23219	804-786-3561
Washington	Department of Health 1112 Southeast Quince Street P.O. Box 47890 Olympia WA 98504	360-753-5871

STATE DEPARTMENTS OF PUBLIC HEALTH Maternal and Child Health Care Contacts		
West Virginia	Division of Maternal and Child Health Department of Health 1411 Virginia Street, E Charleston WV 25301	304-558-5388
	Information Referral:	800-642-8522
	(Regarding eligibility for benefits:) "Client Services" Health and Human Resources Department Capitol Complex, Building 6, Room 607 Charleston WV 25305	304-558-2400
	Information Referral:	800-642-8589
Wisconsin	Health and Social Services Department 1 West Wilson Street Madison WI 53703	608-266-1511
Wyoming	Department of Health Hathaway Building Cheyenne WY 82002	307-777-6186

Chapter 38

Drug Manufacturers' Indigent Programs

For further information, contact:

Pharmaceutical Research and Manufacturers of America (PhRMA)
1100 15 Street, NW
Washington
DC 20005 Tel. 800-PMA-INFO

DRUG MANUFACTURERS' INDIGENT PROGRAMS
Providing Free Prescription Drugs

Drug	Manufacturer - Apply to:	Requirements
Anafranil	Ms. Jackie Laguardia Patient Support Program Administrator **Ciba Pharmaceuticals** 556 Morris Avenue, D-2058 Summit NJ 07901 Tel. 800-257-3273	Eligible if patient is a U.S. resident and "financially unable" to afford this drug. State assistance should be sought first.
Asendin	PARTNERS IN PATIENT CARE™ **Lederle Laboratories** **% Wyeth-Ayerst Laboratories** 555 East Lancaster Avenue St. Davids PA 19087 Tel. 800-568-9938	Available to "Financially indigent" outpatients who are neither eligible for Medicaid nor covered by drugs insurance.

DRUG MANUFACTURERS' INDIGENT PROGRAMS

Providing Free Prescription Drugs

Drug	Manufacturer - Apply to:	Requirements
Desyrel	Patient Assistance Program **Bristol-Myers Squibb** 2400 West Lloyd Expressway Mail Code R-22 Evansville IN 47721 Tel. 800-437-0994	Free to U.S. residents who meet financial criteria of program and who are not eligible for drug coverage elsewhere.
Endep	Ms. Daria Osborne Supervisor, Product Communications Medical Needs Program **Roche Laboratories** 340 Kingsland Street Nutley NJ 07110 Tel. 800-285-4484	"Medically indigent" outpatients who are not reimbursable by another program. Physician determines patient's eligibility.
Ludiomil	Ms. Jackie Laguardia Patient Support Program Administrator **Ciba Pharmaceuticals** 556 Morris Avenue, D-2058 Summit NJ 07901 Tel. 800-257-3273	Eligible if patient is a U.S. resident and "financially unable" to afford this drug. State assistance should be sought first.
Luvox	Patient Assistance Program **Solvay Pharmaceuticals, Inc.** 901 Sawyer Road Marietta GA 30062 Tel. 800-788-9277	Based on a patient's inability to pay, lack of insurance, and ineligibility for Medicaid. Limited to U.S. residents.

DRUG MANUFACTURERS' INDIGENT PROGRAMS

Providing Free Prescription Drugs

Drug	Manufacturer - Apply to:	Requirements
Marplan	Ms. Daria Osborne Supervisor, Product Communications Medical Needs Program **Roche Laboratories** 340 Kingsland Street Nutley NJ 07110 Tel. 800-285-4484	"Medically indigent" outpatients who are not reimbursable by another program. Physician determines whether patient qualifies.
Nardil	The **Parke-Davis** Patient Assistance Program P.O. Box 9945 McLean VA 22102 Tel. 800-755-0120	Eligible if cover is not available elsewhere and financial status meets company guidelines. Patient should call directly for telephone screening and enrollment. Must reapply every six months.
Norpramin	Indigent Patient Program **Hoecht Marion Roussel** P.O. Box 9950 Kansas City MO 64134 Tel. 800-552-3656 816-966-4000	Mainly for patients below federal poverty level and without other cover. Eligibility determined by physician based on patient's level of income.
Pamelor	National Organization for Rare Disorders **Sandoz/NORD Drug Cost Share Program** P.O. Box 8923 New Fairfield CT 06812 Tel. 800-447-6673	Program does not cover this drug.

DRUG MANUFACTURERS' INDIGENT PROGRAMS

Providing Free Prescription Drugs

Drug	Manufacturer - Apply to:	Requirements
Parnate	SB Access to Care Program **SmithKline Beecham Pharmaceuticals** One Franklin Plaza-FP1320 Philadelphia PA 19101 Tel: contact company medical representative.	Very restricted program. Supply limited to six months. Physician determines eligibility and makes application. Patients should not apply.
Paxil	SB Access to Care Program **SmithKline Beecham Pharmaceuticals** One Franklin Plaza-FP1320 Philadelphia PA 19101 Tel. 800-729-4544	Physician determines eligibility and makes application.
Prozac	Lilly Cares Program Administrator Dista Products Division **Eli Lilly and Company** Lilly Corporate Center P.O. Box 9105 McLean VA 22102 Tel. 800-545-6962	Eligibility is based upon patient's "inability to pay" and absence of coverage elsewhere. Replacement drugs not supplied; a fresh application with a new prescription is required.
Serzone	Patient Assistance Program **Bristol-Myers Squibb** 2400 West Lloyd Expressway Mail Code R-22 Evansville IN 47721 Tel. 800-437-0994	Free to U.S. residents who meet financial criteria of program and who are not eligible for drug coverage elsewhere.

DRUG MANUFACTURERS' INDIGENT PROGRAMS

Providing Free Prescription Drugs

Drug	Manufacturer - Apply to:	Requirements
Sinequan (1)	Pfizer Prescription Assistance **Pfizer, Inc.** P.O. Box 25457 Alexandria VA 22313 Tel. 800-646-4455	Free if income below $12,000 (single) or $15,000 (family) and drug coverage is not available elsewhere.
Sinequan (2)	Sharing the Care **Pfizer, Inc.** 13th Floor 235 East 42 Street New York NY 10017 Tel. 800-984-1500	Only patients treated by community, migrant and homeless health centers with in-house pharmacies are eligible. Must be uninsured, below federal poverty line, and ineligible for governmental drug entitlement programs.
Surmontil	Mr. John E. James Professional Services Indigent Patient Program **Wyeth-Ayerst Laboratories** 555 East Lancaster Avenue St. Davids PA 19087 Tel. 800-568-9938	Each case is assessed individually. Eligible if "indigent," i.e., on low or no income and not covered elsewhere.
Tofranil	Ms. Jackie Laguardia Patient Support Program Administrator **Ciba Pharmaceuticals** 556 Morris Avenue, D-2058 Summit NJ 07901 Tel. 800-257-3273	Eligible if patient is a U.S. resident and "financially unable" to afford this drug. State assistance should be sought first.

DRUG MANUFACTURERS' INDIGENT PROGRAMS

Providing Free Prescription Drugs

Drug	Manufacturer - Apply to:	Requirements
Vivactil	The Merck Patient Assistance Program **Merck & Co., Inc.** P.O. Box 4 (WP35-258) West Point PA 19486 Tel. 800-994-2111	Eligible if patient has "financial need" and has exhausted all other means of cover. Must reapply every three months.
Wellbutrin	**Burroughs Wellcome Co.** Patient Assistance Program P.O. Box 52035 Phoenix AZ 85072 Tel. 800-722-9294	Limited to U.S. residents. Must have investigated all other sources of cover. Eligibility based on multiples of the federal poverty guidelines.
Zoloft (1)	Pfizer Prescription Assistance **Pfizer, Inc.** P.O. Box 25457 Alexandria VA 22313 Tel. 800-646-4455	Free if income below $12,000 (single) or $15,000 (family) and patient not eligible for drug coverage elsewhere.
Zoloft (2)	Sharing the Care **Pfizer, Inc.** 13th Floor 235 East 42 Street New York NY 10017 Tel. 800-984-1500	Only patients treated by community, migrant and homeless health centers with in-house pharmacies are eligible. Must be uninsured, below federal poverty line, and ineligible for governmental drug entitlement programs.

Chapter 39

Regional Health Care Financing Administration Offices

Complaints, including denial of emergency treatment facilities, should be made to the Health Standards and Quality Branch of your regional office.

REGIONAL HEALTH CARE FINANCING ADMINISTRATION OFFICES		
Region 1 Connecticut Maine Massachusetts New Hampshire Rhode Island Vermont	Beneficiary Services, Room 2375 JF Kennedy Federal Building Government Center Boston MA 02203	617-565-1188
Region 2 New York New Jersey Puerto Rico Virgin Islands	26 Federal Plaza, Room 3811 New York NY 10278	212-264-4488
Region 3 Delaware Maryland Pennsylvania Virginia West Virginia District of Columbia	3535 Market Street Gateway Building P.O. Box 7760 Philadelphia PA 19101	215-596-1351

REGIONAL HEALTH CARE FINANCING ADMINISTRATION OFFICES

Region 4 Alabama Florida Georgia Kentucky Mississippi North Carolina South Carolina Tennessee	101 Marietta Tower, Suite 701 Atlanta GA 30323	404-331-2329
Region 5 Illinois Indiana Michigan Minnesota Ohio Wisconsin	105 West Adams Street, 15th Floor Chicago IL 60603	312-886-6432
Region 6 Arkansas Louisiana New Mexico Oklahoma Texas	1200 Main Tower Building, Suite 1945 Dallas Texas TX 75202	214-767-6427
Region 7 Iowa Kansas Missouri Nebraska	601 East 12 Street, Room 242 Federal Building Kansas City MO 64106	816-426-5233
Region 8 Colarado Montana North Dakota South Dakota Utah Wyoming	1961 Stout Street Federal Office Building Denver CO 80294	303-844-2111

REGIONAL HEALTH CARE FINANCING ADMINISTRATION OFFICES

Region 9	75 Hawthorne Street	
Arizona	San Francisco	
California	CA 94105	415-744-3502
Hawaii		
Nevada		
Guam		
Pacific Islands Trust Territory		
American Samoa		
Region 10	2201 Sixth Avenue	
Alaska	Blanchard Plaza	
Idaho	Mail Stop RX-40	
Oregon	Seattle	
Washington	WA 98121	206-615-2306

Chapter 40

State Medical Associations

Your State Medical Association can provide you with details of doctors in your area who give some of their time for free or at a reduced charge. Note that these services vary from area to area.

STATE MEDICAL ASSOCIATIONS		
Alabama	19 South Jackson Street Montgomery AL 36104	334-263-6441
Alaska	4107 Laurel Street Anchorage AK 99508	907-562-2662
Arizona	810 West Bethany Home Road Phoenix AZ 85013	602-246-8901
Arkansas	P.O. Box 5776 Little Rock AR 72215	501-224-8967
California	P.O. Box 7690 San Francisco CA 94120	415-541-0900
Colorado	P.O. Box 17550 Denver CO 80217	303-779-5455
Connecticut	160 St. Ronan Street New Haven CT 06511	203-865-0587
Delaware	1925 Lovering Avenue Wilmington DE 19806	302-652-6512

STATE MEDICAL ASSOCIATIONS

District of Columbia	2215 M Street, NW Washington DC 20037	202-466-1800
Florida	760 Riverside Avenue Jacksonville FL 32204	904-356-1571
Georgia	938 Peachtree Street, NE Atlanta GA 30309	404-876-7535
Hawaii	1360 South Bevetania Street Honolulu HI 96814	808-536-7702
Idaho	P.O. Box 2668 Boise ID 83701	208-344-7888
Illinois	20 North Michigan Avenue Suite 700 Chicago IL 60602	312-782-1654
Indiana	322 Canal Walk Indianapolis IN 46202	317-261-2060
Iowa	1001 Grand Avenue West Des Moines IA 50265	515-223-1401
Kansas	623 SW 10 Avenue Topeka KS 66612	913-235-2383
Kentucky	301 North Hurstbourne Parkway Suite 200 Louisville KY 40222	502-426-6200
Louisiana	3501 North Causeway, Suite 800 Metairie LA 70002	504-832-9815
Maine	P.O. Box 190 Manchester ME 04351	207-622-3374

STATE MEDICAL ASSOCIATIONS

Maryland	1211 Cathedral Street Baltimore MD 21201	410-539-0872
Massachusetts	1440 Main Street Waltham MA 02154	617-893-4610
Michigan	120 West Saginaw Street East Lansing MI 48823	517-337-1351
Minnesota	3433 Broadway Street, NE, Suite 300 Minneapolis MN 55413	612-378-1875
Mississippi	735 Riverside Drive Jackson MS 39202	601-354-5433
Missouri	113 Madison Street P.O. Box 1028 Jefferson MO 65102	314-636-5151
Montana	2021 11 Avenue, Suite 1 Helena MT 59601	406-443-4000
Nebraska	233 South 13 Street Suite 1512 Lincoln NE 68508	402-474-4472
Nevada	3660 Baker Lane, Suite 101 Reno NV 89509	702-825-6788
New Hampshire	7 North State Street Concord NH 03301	603-224-1909
New Jersey	2 Princess Road Lawrenceville NJ 08648	609-896-1766

STATE MEDICAL ASSOCIATIONS

New Mexico	7770 Jefferson N.E. Suite #400 Albuquerque NM 87109	505-828-0237
New York	420 Lakeville Road Lake Success NY 11042	516-488-6100
North Carolina	P.O. Box 27167 Raleigh NC 27611	919-833-3836
North Dakota	204 West Thayer Avenue Bismarck ND 58501	701-223-9475
Ohio	1500 Lake Shore Drive Columbus OH 43204	614-486-2401
Oklahoma	601 North West Expressway Oklahoma City OK 73118	405-843-9571
Oregon	5210 Southwest Corbett Avenue Portland OR 97201	503-226-1555
Pennsylvania	777 East Parl Drive P.O. Box 8820 Harrisburg PA 17105	717-558-7750
Rhode Island	106 Francis Street Providence RI 02903	401-331-3207
South Carolina	P.O. Box 11188 Columbia SC 29211	803-798-6207
South Dakota	1323 South Minnesota Avenue Sioux Falls SD 57105	605-336-1965

STATE MEDICAL ASSOCIATIONS

Tennessee	P.O. Box 120909 Nashville TN 37212	615-385-2100
Texas	401 West 15th Street Austin TX 78701	512-370-1300
Utah	540 East 500 South Salt Lake City UT 84102	801-355-7477
Vermont	P.O. Box 1457 Montpelier VT 05601	802-223-7898
Virginia	4205 Dover Road Richmond VA 23221	804-353-2721
Washington	2033 Sixth Avenue, Suite 1100 Seattle WA 98121	206-441-9762
West Virginia	P.O. Box 4106 Charleston WV 25364	304-925-0342
Wisconsin	P.O. Box 1109 Madison WI 53701	608-257-6781
Wyoming	P.O. Drawer 4009 Cheyenne WY 82003	307-635-2424

Chapter 41

Free Information and Advice

Free information and advice about depression is available from Project D/ART (Depression/Awareness, Recognition, Treatment). Contact:

The National Institute of Mental Health (NIMH)
5600 Fishers Lane, Room 7C02
Rockville
MD 20857 Tel. 301-443-4515

Free (or cheap) publications from the NIMH include:

1. A Consumer's Guide to Mental Health Services
   Discusses warning signals of mental health problems, where to go for help, and the kinds of treatment available. Lists other sources of information, including self-help organizations and mutual support groups. (Revised 1994, 21 Pages.)

2. Bipolar Disorder
   (Revised 1993, 12 pages.)

3. D/ART Fact Sheet
   Depression/Awareness, Recognition and Treatment fact sheet. Fold-out brochure.

4. Depression: Patients Get Younger as Rx Options Increase
   Article reprinted from "Medical World News". (August 1990, 7 pages.)

5. Depression: What You Need to Know
   (Revised 1994, 10 pages.)

6. Depression: Effective Treatments are Available
   Fold-out brochure that includes an order form for other free brochures. (Reprinted 1993.)

7. Depressive Illnesses: Treatments Bring New Hope
   An overview of the various depressive illnesses, including causes and symptoms; clinical evaluation and treatment; helpful suggestions for family and friends; and sources of further information. (Revised 1993, 28 pages.)

8. Helpful Facts About Depressive Disorders
(Reprinted 1992, 8 pages.)

9. Helping the Depressed Person Get Treatment
Written in response to requests from concerned family members and friends for help in convincing the depressed person to seek treatment. (1990, 23 pages.)

10. If You're Over 65 and Feeling Depressed ... Treatment Brings New Hope
Many older people believe that their age alone is responsible for feelings of exhaustion, helplessness and worthlessness. This brochure discusses the causes of depression in the older years, symptoms, types of treatment, and where to go for help. (1990, 12 pages.)

11. Information About D/ART and Depression
Provides accurate information about the D/ART Program for organizations interested in developing a program in their community. (1991, 16 pages.)

12. Let's Talk About Depression
Targeted especially to inner city youth, this pamphlet's colorful design and use of celebrity photographs will capture attention. The language, selected for clarity and interest, focuses on depression in a way that young people will understand and identify with. (1991, 6-panel folder.)

13. Plain Talk About Depression
A four-page flyer that discusses types of depression (major depression, dysthymia, cyclothymia, and bipolar disorder), symptoms, diagnostic evaluation and treatment, and how to find help for the depressed person. (Reprinted 1994, 4 pages.)

14. Plain Talk About Handling Stress
(Reprinted 1991, 2 pages.)

15. What to Do When a Friend is Depressed: A Guide for Students
One side of this fold-out brochure offers information on depression and its symptoms and suggests things a young person can do to guide a depressed friend in finding help. The flip side is a poster featuring a relevant quotation. Especially good for health fairs, health clinics and school health units. (1994, 6 panels on one side, poster on the other.)

16. You Are Not Alone
If you suffer from a mental illness, you are not alone. One in five Americans will have a mental illness within their lifetime that is severe enough to require treatment. This pamphlet encourages one to seek help for these highly treatable disorders. It suggests ways to help maintain

good mental health, lists the warning signs of problems, explains the different kinds of mental illnesses, notes available mental health services, and offers resources for additional information.

Publications for the workplace:

17. The Mentally Restored and Work: A Successful Partnership
(1981, 14 pages.)

18. Eight Questions Employers Ask About Hiring the Mentally Restored
(1981, 17 pages.)

19. Managing Depression in the Workpk place
A useful pocket folder that contains information on the D/ART program. (1991.)

20. Poster for Employers: "Not Everyone With Depression Is This Visible"
Treat Depression before it becomes obvious. (Available in two sizes: 16½" x 22" (sent folded) and 8½"x 11".)

21. What to Do When an Employee is Depressed: A Guide for Supervisors
A D/ART program brochure that will enable an employer to recognize the symptoms of depression in an employee and offers suggestions on how to encourage him (her) to seek help. (6-panel folder.)

Publications of professional interest:

22. Approaching the 21st Century: Opportunities for NIMH Neuroscience Research (1988)
A report to Congress from the National Advisory Mental Health Council. It describes the recent advances made by neuroscientists in their search for the causes of mental illnesses, effective treatment and cures. It also describes the accomplishments that can be anticipated during the "Decade of the Brain." (1988, 105 pages.)

23. ECA Update
This is a table showing the prevalence of mental disorders during a one-month period and during a year, as determined by a multisite epidemiological and health services research survey conducted between 1980–1984. The survey was supported by NIMH and called the Epidemiologic Catchment Area (ECA) study. (August 1993.)

24. National Plan for Research on Child and Adolescent Mental Disorders
Submitted to the Congress by the National Advisory Mental Health Council, this plan addresses the status of research concerning mental disorders in young Americans and the steps that must be taken to free our youth of the costly, tragic burdens of mental illness. (1990, 64 pages.)

25. Psychopharmacology Bulletin (Quarterly Journal)
This publication emphasizes rapid, informal dissemination of recent research findings that have not previously appeared in the more formal literature. The first two issues each year focus on the vast array of materials presented at the annual New Clinical Drug Evaluation Unit (NCDEU) meeting. The third issue is devoted to the publication of summaries of papers presented at the annual American College of Neuropsycopharmacology meeting. The remaining issue is devoted to proceedings of NIMH workshops, reviews, and special issues organized around a central theme.

26. Suicide Facts

Suicide is the eighth leading cause of death in the United States. Additional facts about suicide, the risk factors associated with suicide, data on attempted suicides, and prevention information are included in this updated fact sheet. (1994, 1 page.)

27. The Value of Psychiatric Treatment: Its Efficacy in Severe Mental Disorders
An issue of the NIMH "Psychopharmacology Bulletin," this volume provides a clear and concise summary of the scientific data on treatment efficacy for severe mental illnesses (schizophrenia, bipolar disorder, major depression, panic disorder and obsessive-compulsive disorder) as well as mental illness in geriatric patients and in children and adolescents. This volume is an excellent resource for information on the status of the field of psychiatric treatment research for the severely mentally ill. (Psychopharmacology Bulletin, Volume 29(4), 1993. Reprinted 1994, 132 pages.)

Publications in Spanish:

28. Datos Utiles Sobre Enfermedadas Depresivas
(Helpful Facts About Depressive Disorders.)

29. Depresion/Advertencia, Reconocimiento, Tratamiento
(D/ART) Fact Sheet

30. Depresion: Lo Que Usted Necesita Saber
(Depression: What You Need to Know.)

31. La Depresion: Existen Tratamientos Eficaces
(Depression: Effective Treatments are Available.)

32. No Estas Solo: Datos Acerca de Salud Mental y Enfermedades
(You Are Not Alone: Facts About Mental Health and Mental Illness.)

33. Platica Franca Sobre La Tension
(Plain Talk About Stress.)

34. Una Guia Sobre Servicios De Salud Mental Para Los Consumidores
(A Consumer's Guide to Mental Health Services.)

Information specific to depression and the elderly can also be obtained from:

The National Institute on Aging (NIA)
Building 31, Room 5C27
Bethesda
MD 20892 Tel. 301-496-1752

Free (or cheap) publications from the NIA include:

35. Diagnosis and Treatment of Depression in Late Life
Alerting both the professional and the general public to the seriousness of depression in late life, this report discusses epidemiology, pathogenesis, pathophysiology, prevention and treatment. Among its conclusions, it finds that the highest rates of depression occur in nursing and residential homes whose staff are generally not equipped to recognize or treat depressed patients. (A consensus statement by the National Institute of Health Consensus Development Conference November 4–6, 1991, Volume 9, Number 3. 26 pages.)

36. Perspectives in Health Promotion and Aging (Quarterly Journal)
This publication is a service of the National Eldercare Institute on Health Promotion and the American Association of Retired Persons (AARP). It promotes effective approaches to healthy behaviors and practices for the elderly, including mental wellness.

37. Fact Sheet: How Physical and Mental Health Interact in Older Persons
(1991, 2 pages.)

38. Fact Sheet: Mental Health and Aging; Scientific Discoveries and Prospects
(undated, 2 pages.)

39. Fact Sheet: Depression in the Elderly
(1989, 5 pages.)

Videos, tapes, computer software, and other audiovisuals about depression can be obtained from your local library by means of an interlibrary loan from:

The National Library of Medicine
8600 Rockville Pike
Bethesda
MD 20894 Tel. 800-272-4787

Vidoes available include the following titles:

40. Downtime: Understanding Clinical Depression in the Worksite
At the worksite supervisors and coworkers can play an important role in recognizing early warning signs. Dick Cavett narrates the tale of two employees who were diagnosed with clinical depression. Their supervisors relate their stories of treatment, recovery, and return to work. (Produced by the Depressive and Related Affective Disorders Association (DRADA) in cooperation with the Wellness Councils of America (WELCOA).)

41. Overcoming Depression
Psychotherapy is illustrated with case studies. (Produced by the Institute for Rational-Emotive Therapy, New York.)

42. Treating Depression: Preventing Suicide
(Produced by the University of Wisconsin Hospital and Clinics.)

43. Treating Depression in the Elderly
(Produced by Marshfield Clinic, Wisconsin.)

44. Diagnosis and Treatment of Anxiety and Depression in the Elderly
The diagnostical complexities of depression are examined, and the contrasting symptoms of depression, anxiety, insomnia and dementia are discussed. Pharmacologic and other somatic treatments are explored. (Produced by Marshfield Clinic, Wisconsin.)

45. Newer Treatments for Depression
Dr. James Jefferson reviews newer drug treatments and their side effects. (Produced by Marshfield Clinic, Wisconsin.)

46. Reducing Resident Depression: Assessment and Intervention
Depression in a nursing home environment is examined. The difficulty in telling major depression apart from natural sadness and demoralization due to life circumstances is shown. Identifying and managing symptoms of depression are explained. (Produced by the University of Maryland at Baltimore.)

47. Teen and Childhood Depression
Even psychologists sometimes fail to diagnose severe depression in their own children. This video describes the common symptoms of depression: crying, withdrawal, over- or undereating, oversleeping or insomnia, concentration and memory problems, getting no pleasure out of life, and, in the extreme cases, suicide. Possible causes are examined, including biological and environmental factors such as child abuse. Treatments are discussed. (Produced by Films for the Humanities and Sciences, Princeton, New Jersey.)

48. Women and Disease
This program examines the lack of medical research conducted on women, resulting in poorer treatments in the areas of heart disease, depression and alcoholism. (Produced by Films for the Humanities and Sciences, Princeton, New Jersey, in conjunction with the Dartmouth-Hitchcock Medical Center.)

49. Atypical Depression
(Produced by the Medical University of South Carolina, Health Communications Network.)

50. Depression: New Treatment Options
This video describes depression and how it envelopes and dominates a person's life. This devastating disorder has affected people throughout the ages, some of whom go on to make enormous contributions to society. Unfortunately, some twelve per cent eventually commit suicide when their illness is untreated. (Produced by Marshfield Clinic, Wisconsin.)

51. Depression: The Storm Within
A general discussion of depression. (Produced by the American Psychiatric Association.)

52. Depression
Five brief public service announcements. (Produced by the National Institute of Mental Health.)

53. What About Prozac?
Drug therapy and therapeutic use of fluoxetine, marketed as prozac. (Produced by Ambrose Video Publishing.)

54. Crying for Happiness
Therapy, care and patient participation in overcoming depression (Produced by Skyworks Charitable Foundation, Canada.)

55. Depression and the Elderly
Diagnosis and therapy. (Produced by Fairview Audiovisuals, Cleveland, Ohio.)

56. ECT in the Treatment of Major Depression
Use and tends of electroconvulsive therapy in treating major depression. (Produced by the Medical University of South Carolina, Health Communications Network.)

57. Geriatric Psychopharmacology: An Update
(Produced by the Medical University of South Carolina, Health Communications Network.)

58. Management of Depression in Childhood
Depression in infancy, childhood and adolescence. (Produced by Marshfield Clinic, Wisconsin.)

59. Psychotherapy of Depression
(Produced by the Medical University of South Carolina, Health Communications Network.)

60. Coping with Aging
(Produced by Marshfield Clinic, Wisconsin.)

61. Diagnosis of Depression in Adolescents
Since early intervention can prevent the emotional, physical, and social dysfunctions often associated with depression, early recognition is stressed. A review is made of the diagnostic symptoms that mask depression such as behavioral problems, substance abuse, and antisocial behavior. (Produced by the Network for Continuing Medical Education, Secaucus, New Jersey.)

62. Manic Depression: The Agony and The Ecstacy
A description of manic depression, diagnosis, treatments, and drug therapy. (Produced by Mending the Mind, Waco, Texas.)

63. Teen Suicide and Depression
Includes a 20-page guide. (Produced by the Ridgeview Institute, Atlanta, Georgia.)

Cassette tape recordings available include the following titles:

64. Panic Disorder, Agoraphobia, and Depression,
31 color slides, a sound cassette and a guide. (Produced by the Ohio Medical Education Network, Columbus.)

65. Depression and Suicide: Multidisciplinary Assessment and Treatment
A biological, psychological and social model for understanding and treating depressive episodes and long-term conditions, including suicidal

tendencies. (Produced by the American Healthcare Institute, Silver Spring, Maryland.)

66. Manic Depression: Voices of an Illness
Narrated by acclaimed actress Patty Duke, who has lived through and overcome this illness. (Produced by Lichtenstein Creative Media, New York.)

67. Maternal Depression and Early Child Development
(Produced by the World Association for Infant Psychiatry and Allied Disciplines, Fifth World Congress, 1992, Chicago.)

68. Mood Altering Agents
Pharmacology, use and side effects of tricyclic antidepressants, MAOI antidepressants and lithium. (Produced by the Menniger Foundation, Topeka, Kansas.)

69. Postpartum Depression: Therapeutic Teamwork Between Psychiatry and Pediatrics
(Produced by the World Association for Infant Psychiatry and Allied Disciplines, Fifth World Congress, 1992, Chicago.)

70. Postpartum Depression: Research and Clinical Perspectives
(Produced by the World Association for Infant Psychiatry and Allied Disciplines, Fifth World Congress, 1992, Chicago.)

71. Special Problems in the Psychotherapy of Depression
(Produced by the American Psychoanalytic Association, Chicago.)

72. Depression: Diagnosis and Treatment
A thorough investigation including the following topics: introduction, atypical depression, non-responding depression, chronic depression, depression and personality disorders, delusional, depression, and depression and suicide. A 53 page guide is included. (Produced by Guildford Publications, New York.)

73. Depression in Childhood and Adolescence
Includes 25 color slides, a sound cassette, and a guide. (Produced by Ohio Medical Education Network, Columbus.)

Chapter 42

Self-Help Organizations

The information below has been extracted from the "Self-Help Sourcebook" (fifth edition © 1995), compiled and edited by Barbara J. White and Edward J. Madara. It is reprinted by permission of the American Self-Help Clearinghouse, Northwest Covenant Medical Center, 25 Pocono Road, Denville, NJ 07834. Further information can be obtained by purchasing this useful book.

SELF-HELP ORGANIZATIONS FOR DEPRESSION AND RELATED DISORDERS	
For those with the illness:	
Children's and Youth Emotions Anonymous P.O. Box 4245 St. Paul MN 55104 Tel. 612-647-9712	Twelve-step program to help youth develop healthy emotions, attitudes and habits. Youth groups led by adult members of Emotions Anonymous (see below).
Depressed Anonymous Depressed Self-Help Services, Inc. P.O. Box 17471 Louisville KY 40217 Tel. 502-569-1989	Twelve-step program to give depressed persons hope and belief in recovery. Newsletter, phone support, information and referrals, pen friends, workshops, conferences and seminars. Information packet ($5).

SELF-HELP ORGANIZATIONS FOR DEPRESSION AND RELATED DISORDERS	
For those with the illness:	
Depression After Delivery P.O. Box 1282 Morrisville PA 19067 Tel. 800-944-4773 Tel. 215-295-3994	Support and information for women who have suffered from postpartum depression. Telephone support in most states, newsletter, group development guidelines, pen friends, and conferences.
Depressives Anonymous 329 East 62 Street New York NY 10021 Tel. 212-689-2600	Helps anxious and depressed people change troublesome behavior patterns and attitudes about living. Professional involvement. Newsletter, group development guidelines.
Depression and Related Affective Disorders (DRADA) Meyer Building, 3-181 600 North Wolfe Street Baltimore MD 21287 Tel. 410-955-4647	Alleviates suffering arising from depression and manic-depression by providing education, information, supporting research, and assisting self-help groups. Newsletter.
Emotional Health Anonymous P.O. Box 429 Glendale CA 91202 Tel. 818-240-3215	Twelve-step program to solve common problems of mental health. Fellowship of people who meet to share experiences, hopes, and strengths. Newsletter.
Emotions Anonymous P.O. Box 4245 St. Paul MN 55104 Tel. 612-647-9712	Twelve-step program to gain better emotional health. Fellowship of people sharing experiences, hopes and strengths. Correspondence program for those who cannot attend meetings.

SELF-HELP ORGANIZATIONS FOR DEPRESSION AND RELATED DISORDERS	
For those with the illness:	
GROW in America, Inc. 2403 West Springfield Avenue P.O. Box 3367 Champaign IL 61826 Tel. 217-352-6989	Twelve-step mutual help program to provide know-how for avoiding and recovering from a breakdown. Caring and sharing community to attain maturity and personal responsibility. Newsletter.
International Association for Clear Thinking (IACT) P.O. Box 1011 Appleton WI 54912 Tel. 800-236-8311 (in WI) Tel. 414-739-8311 (elsewhere)	For those interested in living their lives more effectively and satisfactorily. Uses principles of clear thinking and self-counselling. Newsletter, group handbook, audio tapes, facilitator leadership training, self-help materials.
National Depressive and Manic-Depressive Association (NDMDA) 730 North Franklin Street, Suite 501 Chicago IL 60610 Tel. 800-826-3632 Tel. 312-642-0049	Mutual support and information for sufferers and families. Public education on illness and availability of treatment. Annual conferences, chapter development guidelines.
National Organization for Seasonal Affective Disorder (NOSAD) P.O. Box 40133 Washington DC 20016 Tel. 301-762-0768	Information and education about the causes, nature and treatment of seasonal affective disorder (SAD). Encourages development of services to patients and families, and research into causes and treatment.

SELF-HELP ORGANIZATIONS FOR DEPRESSION AND RELATED DISORDERS	
For those with the illness:	
Neurotics Anonymous Route 1, Box 12 Casa AR 72025 Tel. 501-233-6651	Twelve-step program to help mentally and emotionally disturbed people recover from their illness and maintain their recovery. Information, phone support, newsletter.
Reclamation, Inc. HC4, Box 254 Blanco Texas TX 78606 Tel. 210-833-4946	Alliance of former mental patients helping to eliminate stigma of mental illness. Helps with social, employment and housing problems. Newsletter.
Recoveries Anonymous P.O. Box 1212 Hewitt Square Station East Northport NY 11731 Tel. 516-261-1212	Fellowship focussing on spiritual solutions of the twelve-step program. Geared to those who have been unsuccessful so far in finding a recovery.
Recovery, Inc. 802 North Dearborn Street Chicago IL 60610 Tel. 312-337-5661	Community mental health organization offering a self-help method of will training, a system of techniques for controlling temperamental behavior, and changing attitudes towards nervous symptoms and fears. Publication "Recovery Reporter" for members.

SELF-HELP ORGANIZATIONS FOR DEPRESSION AND RELATED DISORDERS	
For families and friends:	
Federation of Families for Children's Mental Health 1021 Prince Street Alexandria VA 22314 Tel. 703-684-7710	Attends to needs of children and youth with emotional, behavioral or mental disorders; and their families. Run by parents. Information and advocacy, newsletter, conferences.
National Alliance for the Mentally Ill (NAMI) 200 North Glebe Road, Suite 1015 Arlington VA 22203 Tel. 800-950-NAMI Tel. 703-524-7600	Network of self-help groups for relatives of the seriously mentally ill. Emotional and educational support. Bi-monthly newsletter, affiliate development guidelines.

SELF-HELP ORGANIZATIONS FOR DEPRESSION AND RELATED DISORDERS	
Related groups:	
Anxiety Disorders Association of America 6000 Executive Boulevard, Suite 513 Rickville MD 20852 Tel. 301-231-9350	Promotes welfare of people with phobias and anxieties. For consumers, health care professionals and concerned others. National Membership Directory. Self-Help Group Directory. Newsletters.
Fear of Success Anonymous 16161 Ventura Boulevard, Suite 727 Encino CA 91436 Tel. 818-907-3953	Twelve-step program to overcome fears, avoid self-sabotaging behavior and take action. For people committed to obtaining and enjoying the benefits of success in all areas of our lives.
Obsessive-Compulsive Anonymous (OCA) P.O. Box 215 New Hyde Park NY 11040 Tel. 516-741-4901	Twelve-step program to assist people with obsessive-compulsive disorder.
Phobics Anonymous P.O. Box 1180 Palm Springs CA 92263 Tel. 619-322-COPE	Twelve-step program to recover from anxiety and panic disorders. Fellowship for sufferers.

Chapter 43

Self-Help Clearinghouses

Contact one of these clearinghouses to find out the names of all the self-help groups operating in your locality which deal in your area of interest.

The information below has been extracted from the "Self-Help Sourcebook" (fifth edition © 1995), compiled and edited by Barbara J. White and Edward J. Madara. It is reprinted by permission of the American Self-Help Clearinghouse, Northwest Covenant Medical Center, 25 Pocono Road, Denville, NJ 07834. Further information can be obtained by purchasing this useful book.

SELF-HELP CLEARINGHOUSES
(* = Statewide Referrals)

State	Institution	
Nationwide	American Self-Help Clearinghouse % Northwest Covenant Medical Center 25 Pocono Road Denville NJ 07834	Tel. 201-625-7101
Information	National Self-Help Clearinghouse City University of New York Graduate School and University Center 25 West 43rd Street, Room 620 New York NY 10036	Tel. 212-354-8525
Alabama	—	
Alaska	—	
Alberta, Canada	Family Life Education Council 233 12 Avenue SW Calgary, Alberta T2R 0G9	Tel. 403-262-1117

SELF-HELP CLEARINGHOUSES

(* = Statewide Referrals)

State	Institution	
Arizona	Rainy day People P.O. Box 472 Scottsdale AZ 85252	Tel. 602-231-0868
Arkansas	Arkansas Helpline P.O. Box 9028 Jonesboro AR 72403	Tel. 501-932-5555
British Columbia, Canada	Self-Help Resource Association of British Columbia 175 Broadway Vancouver, British Columbia V5Y 1P4	Tel. 604-876-6086
California (Davis)	Mental Health Association of Yolo County P.O. Box 447 Davis CA 95617	Tel. 916-756-8181
California (Los Angeles*)	California Self-Help Center % University of California at Los Angeles Psychiatry Department 405 Hilgard Avenue Los Angeles CA 90024	Tel. 800-222-5465 Tel. 310-825-1799
California (Modesto)	Friends Network 800 Scenic Drive Modesto CA 95350	209-558-7454
California (Riverside)	Riverside Mental Health Association 3763 Arlington Avenue, Suite 103 Riverside CA 92506	Tel. 909-684-6051
California (Sacramento)	Mental Health Association 8912 Volunteer Lane, Suite 210 Sacramento CA 95826	Tel. 916-368-3100

SELF-HELP CLEARINGHOUSES

(* = Statewide Referrals)

State	Institution	
California (San Diego)	Self-Help Connection % Mental Health Association San Diego County 1202 Morena Boulevard, Suite 203 San Diego CA 92110	Tel. 619-275-0607
California (San Francisco)	Bay Area Self-Help Center % Mental Health Association 2398 Pine Street San Francisco CA 94115	Tel. 415-921-4044
Colorado	—	
Connecticut	Connecticut Self-Help/Mutual Support Network Consultation Center 389 Whitney Avenue New Haven CT 06511	Tel. 203-789-7645
Delaware	—	
District of Columbia (and area surrounding)	Self-Help Clearinghouse of Greater Washington % Mental Health Association of Northern Virginia 7630 Little River Turnpike, Suite 206 Annandale VA 22003	Tel. 703-941-5465
Florida	—	
Georgia	—	
Hawaii	—	
Idaho	—	
Illinois (Champaign)	Champaign Self-Help Center % Family Service of Champaign County 405 South State Street Champaign IL 61820	Tel. 217-352-0099
Illinois (Chicago*)	Illinois Self-Help Coalition % Wright College, Room 244 3400 North Austin Street Chicago IL 60634	Tel. 312-481-8837

SELF-HELP CLEARINGHOUSES

(* = Statewide Referrals)

State	Institution	
Illinois (Chicago*)	Illinois Self-Help Center % Mental Health Association in Illinois 150 Wacher Drive, Suite 900 Chicago IL 60606	Tel. 708-291-0085
Illinois (Decatur)	Macon County Support Group Network % Macon County Health Department 1221 East Condit Street Decatur IL 62521	Tel. 217-429-4357
Indiana	—	
Iowa	Iowa Pilot Parents Self-Help Clearinghouse 33 North 12 Street P.O. Box 1151 Fort Dodge IA 50501	Tel. 800-952-4777 Tel. 515-576-5870
Kansas	Self-Help Network of Kansas Campus Box 34 Wichita State University 1845 Fairmont Street Wichita KS 67260	Tel. 800-445-0116 Tel. 316-689-3843
Kentucky	—	
Louisiana	—	
Maine	—	
Manitoba, Canada	Winnpeg Self-Help Resource Clearinghouse NorWest Coope and Health Center 103-61 Tyndall Avenue Winnipeg, Manitoba R2X 2T4	Tel. 204-589-5500 Tel. 204-633-5955
Maryland (see District of Columbia)	—	

SELF-HELP CLEARINGHOUSES

(* = Statewide Referrals)

State	Institution	
Massachusetts	Massachusetts Clearinghouse of Mutual Help Groups % Massachusetts Cooperative Extension System Department of Consumer Studies 113 Skinner Hall University of Massachusetts Amherst MA 01003	Tel. 413-545-2313
Michigan (Benton Harbor)	Southwest Michigan/Northern Indiana Center for Self-Help % Riverwood Center P.O. Box 547 Benton Harbor MI 49023	Tel. 800-336-0341 Tel. 616-925-0594
Michigan (Lansing*)	Michigan Self-Help Clearinghouse 106 West Allegan Street, Suite 210 Lansing MI 48933	Tel. 800-777-5556 Tel. 517-484-7373
Minnesota	—	
Mississippi	—	
Missouri (Kansas City)	Mental Health Association of Kansas City 7611 State Line Road, Suite 230 Kansas City MO 64105	Tel. 816-822-7272
Missouri (St. Louis)	St. Louis Self-Help Clearinghouse % Greater St. Louis Mental Health Association 1905 South Grand Boulevard St. Louis MO 63104	Tel. 314-773-1399
Montana	—	
Nebraska	Nebraska Self-Help Information Services 1601 Euclid Avenue Lincoln NE 68502	Tel. 402-476-9668
Nevada	—	

SELF-HELP CLEARINGHOUSES

(* = Statewide Referrals)

State	Institution
New Hampshire	New Hampshire HELPLINE 2 Industrial Park Drive Concord NH 03301 Tel. 800-852-3388 Tel. 603-225-9000
New Jersey	New Jersey Self-Help Clearinghouse % Northwest Covenant Medical Center 25 Pocono Road Denville NJ 07834 Tel. 201-625-7101
New Mexico	—
New York (New York City)	New York Self-Help Center 120 West 57 Street New York NY 10019 Tel. 212-586-5770
New York	Other clearinghouses:
(Amsterdam)	Montgomery County Self-Help Clearinghouse Tel. 518-842-1900 ext. 351 or 279
(Binghampton)	Broome County Self-Help Clearinghouse Tel. 607-771-8888
(Brooklyn)	Brooklyn Self-Help Clearinghouse Tel. 718-875-1420
(Buffalo)	Erie County Self-Help Clearinghouse Tel. 716-886-1242
(Cobleskill)	Schoharie County Community Action Program Tel. 518-234-2568
(Corning)	Stueben County HELPLINE Tel. 800-346-2211/607-936-4114
(Goshen)	Helpline/Rapeline of Orange, Ulster and Sullivan Counties Tel. 800-832-1200/914-294-7411
(Ithaca)	Tompkins County Mental Health Association Tel. 607-273-9250
(Kingston)	Ulster County Mental Health Association Tel. 914-339-9090
(Johnstown)	Fulton County HealthLink Tel. 518-736-1120

SELF-HELP CLEARINGHOUSES

(* = Statewide Referrals)

State	Institution
New York	Other clearinghouses (cont.):
(Lockport)	Niagra Self-Help Clearinghouse Tel. 716-433-3780
(Mechanicville)	Mechanicville Area Community Services Center Tel. 518-664-8322
(New City)	Rockland Self-Help Clearinghouse Tel. 914-639-7400
(Olean)	Cattaraugus County Self-Help Clearinghouse Tel. 716-372-5800
(Poughkeepsie)	United Way Self-Help Clearinghouse of Duchess County Tel. 914-473-1500
(Potsdam)	Reachout of St. Lawrence County Tel. 315-265-2422
(Rochester)	Monroe County Clearinghouse for Self-Help Groups Tel. 716-256-0590
(Rome)	Rome Volunteer Action Center Tel. 315-336-5644
(Schenectady)	Schenectady Information Line Tel. 518-374-2244
(Syracuse)	Syracuse HELPLINE Information and Referral Service Tel. 315-474-7011
(Warsaw)	Wyoming County Chapter American Cross Tel. 716-786-0540
(White Plains)	Westchester Self-Help Clearinghouse Tel. 914-949-6301
North Carolina	Mecklenberg County SupportWorks Self-Help Clearinghouse 1018 East Boulevard, Suite 5 Charlotte NC 28203 Tel. 704-331-9500
North Dakota	Fargo Hot Line P.O. Box 447 Fargo ND 58107 Tel. 701-293-6462

SELF-HELP CLEARINGHOUSES

(* = Statewide Referrals)

State	Institution
Nova Scotia, Canada	The Self-Help Connection of Nova Scotia Mental Health Association 63 King Street Dartmouth, Nova Scotia B2Y 2R7 Tel. 902-466-2011
Ohio (Dayton)	Greater Dayton Self-Help Clearinghouse % Family Services Association 184 Salem Avenue Dayton OH 45406 Tel. 513-225-3004
Ohio (Toledo)	Greater Toledo Self-Help Network % Harbor Behavioral Health Care 123 22 Street Toledo OH 43624 Tel. 419-241-6191
Oklahoma	—
Ontario, Canada	Clearinghouse of Metropolitan Toronto 40 Orchard View Boulevard, Suite 219 Toronto, Ontario M4R 1B9 Tel. 416-487-4355
Oregon	Northwest Regional Self-Help Clearinghouse 619 Southwest 11 Street, Room 300 Portland OR 97205 Tel. 503-222-5555
Pennsylvania (Pittsburgh)	Self-Help Group Network of the Pittsburgh Area 1323 Forbes Avenue, Suite 200 Pittsburgh PA 15219 Tel. 412-261-5363
Pennsylvania (Scranton)	Self-Help Information Network Exchange 538 Spruce Street, Suite 420 Scranton PA 18503 Tel. 717-961-1234
Puerto Rico	—
Rhode Island	—

SELF-HELP CLEARINGHOUSES

(* = Statewide Referrals)

State	Institution
South Carolina	Midland Area Support Group Network % Lexington Medical Center 2720 Sunset Boulevard West Columbia SC 26169 Tel. 803-791-2800
South Dakota	—
Tennessee (Knoxville)	Knox County Support Group Clearinghouse % Mental Health Association of Greater Knoxville 6712 Kingston Pike, Suite 203 Knoxville TN 37919 Tel. 615-584-9125
Tennessee (Memphis)	Memphis and Shelby Counties Self-Help Clearinghouse % Mental Health Association 2400 Poplar Avenue, Suite 410 Memphis TN 38112 Tel. 901-323-0858
Texas (Austin*)	Texas Self-Help Clearinghouse % Mental Health Association in Texas 8401 Shoal Creek Boulevard Austin TX 78757 Tel. 512-454-3706
Texas (Dallas)	Dallas Self-Help Clearinghouse % Mental Health Association of Greater Dallas 2929 Carlisle Street, Suite 350 Dallas TX 75204 Tel. 214-871-2420
Texas (Fort Worth)	Tarrant County Self-Help Clearinghouse % Mental Health Association of Tarrant County 3136 West 4 Street Fort Worth TX 76107 Tel. 817-335-5405
Texas (Houston)	Houston Area Self-Help Clearinghouse % Mental Health Association in Houston and Harris County 2211 Norfolk, Suite 810 Houston TX 77098 Tel. 713-522-5161

SELF-HELP CLEARINGHOUSES

(* = Statewide Referrals)

State	Institution	
Texas (San Antonio)	Mental Health Information Center % Mental Health Association in Greater San Antonio 901 North East Loop 410, Suite 704 San Antonio TX 78209	Tel. 210-826-2288
Utah	Information and Referral Center 1025 South 700 West Salt Lake City UT 84106	Tel. 801-978-3333
Vermont	—	
Virginia (see District of Columbia)	—	

Bibliography

Adams, Andrea. *Bullying at Work: How to Confront and Overcome it.* London: Virago Press, 1992.

Balch, James F., M.D., and Phyllis A. Balch. *Prescription for Nutritional Healing*. Garden City Park, New York: Avery Publishing Group, 1990.

Burns, David D., M.D. *Feeling Good: The New Mood Therapy.* New York: Avon Books, 1992.

Columbia University College of Physicians and Surgeons. *The Columbia University College of Physicians and Surgeons Complete Home Guide to Mental Health.* Ed. Frederic I. Kass, M.D., John M. Oldham, M.D., Herbert Pardes, M.D., and Lois B. Morris. New York: Henry Holt and Company, 1992.

Copeland, Mary Ellen. *The Depression Workbook: A Guide for Living with Depression and Manic Depression.* Oakland, California: New Harbinger Publications, 1992.

DePaulo, J. Raymond, Jr., M.D., and Keith Russell Ablow, M.D. *How to Cope with Depression*. Baltimore: John Hopkins University Press, 1989.

Dowling, Collette. *You Mean I Don't Have to Feel This Way?: New Help for Depression, Anxiety, and Addiction*. New York: Scribner, 1991.

Engler, Jack, and Daniel Goleman. *The Consumer's Guide to Psychotherapy.* New York: Simon and Schuster/Fireside, 1992.

Fieve, Ronald R., M.D. *Prozac: Questions and Answers for Patients, Family, and Physicians*. New York: Avon Books, 1994.

Giller, Robert, M.D., and Kathy Matthews. *Natural Prescriptions: Dr. Robert Giller's Natural Treatments and Vitamin Therapies for over 100 Common Ailments.* New York: Carol Southern Books, 1994.

Goldberg, Ivan K., M.D. *Questions and Answers about Depression and its Treatment: A Consultation with a Leading Psychiatrist.* Philadelphia: Charles Press, 1993.

Gorman, Jack M., M.D. *The Essential Guide to Psychiatric Drugs.* Updated ed. New York: St. Martin's Press, 1992.

Greist, John H., M.D., and James W Jefferson, M.D. *Depression and its Treatment: A Layman's Guide by Two Leading Psychiatrists to Help You Understand and Cope with America's Number One Health Problem.* New York: Warner Books, 1994.

Griffith, H. Winter, M.D. *Complete Guide to Prescription and Non-Prescription Drugs.* Rev. ed. New York: Body Press, Berkley Publishing Group, 1994.

Homeopathy for the Family. 13th ed. London: Wigmore Publications Ltd., 1994.

Jamison, K. Redfield, M.D. *The Unquiet Mind.* New York: Random House, 1995.

Klein, Herbert E., ed., *Psychotherapy Finances.* Jupiter, Florida: Ridgewood Financial Institute, Inc., 1995.

Kline, Nathan S., M.D. *From Sad to Glad.* Rev. ed. New York: Ballantine Books, 1993.

Meeks, John E., M.D. *High Times/Low Times: The Many Faces of Adolescent Depression.* Washington, D.C., PIA Press, 1988.

Naifeh, Steven and Gregory White Smith. *The Best Doctors in America.* Aiken, South Carolina: Woodward/White, Inc., 1992.

Norden, Michael J., M.D. *Beyond Prozac; Brain-toxic Lifestyles, Natural Antidotes, and New Generation Antidepressants.* New York: Harper-Collins Publishers, 1995.

Papalos, Demitri F., M.D., and Janice Papalos. *Overcoming Depression.* New York, Harper and Row, 1988

People's Medical Society, comp. *Dial 800 for Health.* Allentown, Pennsylvania: People's Medical Society, 1993.

Preston, John. *You can Beat Depression: A Guide to Recovery.* San Luis Obispo, California: Impact Publishers, 1992

Robinson, Rita. *Survivors of Suicide.* Van Nuys, California: Newcastle Publishing Co., 1989.

Smith, Hugh M. *Depressed? Here is a Way Out.* London: HarperCollins Publishers, 1991.

Thorne, Julia, and Larry Rothstein. *You are Not Alone: Words of Experience and Hope for the Journey through Depression.* New York: HarperCollins Publishers, 1993.

White, Barbara J., and Edward J. Madara, eds. and comps. *The Self-Help Sourcebook.* 4th ed. Denville, New Jersey: St. Clares–Riverside Medical Center, 1992.

Wright, John W., and Linda Sunshine. *The Best Hospitals in America.* Detroit, Michigan: Visible Ink Press, 1995.

Wurtzel, Elizabeth. *Prozac Nation: Young and Depressed in America.* New York: Riverhead Books, Berkley Publishing Group, 1995.

Index

Order Form

☎ **To order by credit card call:**

1-800-444-2524 (toll-free)
1-941-758-8094 (international orders)
1-941-753-9396 (fax)

☒ **Or send a check or money order to:**

BookWorld Services, Inc.
1933 Whitfield Park Loop
Sarasota, FL 34243

Please send me _____ copies of *Conquer Depression Now; From Sad to Glad at Home, School, and Work* at $14.95 each. I understand that I may return any books for a full refund—for any reason, no questions asked.

Name:____

Address:____

City:_____________________________ State:____ Zip:__________

Sales tax: Florida residents please add appropriate sales tax.

Shipping: Book rate: $3.95 for the first book. Add $2 for each additional book. Delivery takes 7–10 working days. UPS rate: telephone to obtain current price.

Payment: ☐ Check ☐ Credit card

☐ VISA ☐ MASTERCARD ☐ AMEX ☐ DISCOVER

Card number:_______________________________________

Name on card:_____________________________ Exp. date:_______

Call *toll-free* and order now

Order Form

☎ **To order by credit card call:**

1-800-444-2524 (toll-free)
1-941-758-8094 (international orders)
1-941-753-9396 (fax)

☒ **Or send a check or money order to:**

BookWorld Services, Inc.
1933 Whitfield Park Loop
Sarasota, FL 34243

Please send me _____ copies of *Conquer Depression Now; From Sad to Glad at Home, School, and Work* at $14.95 each. I understand that I may return any books for a full refund—for any reason, no questions asked.

Name:____

Address:______________________________________

City:________________________ State:____ Zip:_________

Sales tax: Florida residents please add appropriate sales tax.

Shipping: Book rate: $3.95 for the first book. Add $2 for each additional book. Delivery takes 7–10 working days. UPS rate: telephone to obtain current price.

Payment: ☐ Check ☐ Credit card

☐ VISA ☐ MASTERCARD ☐ AMEX ☐ DISCOVER

Card number:___________________________________

Name on card:______________________ Exp. date:_______

Call *toll-free* and order now